D1490671

The Asperger's Syndrome Survival Guide

Plus the following bonus guides:

How To Be Your Child's Best Advocate
Making the Transition to Adulthood
Helping Your Aspergers Child Cope with the Holiday Season
The Aspergers Survey of Parents and Professionals

Craig Kendall

Dedicated to my
wonderful family
and to all who
desire longer life so
they can serve more

The Asperger's Syndrome Survival Guide

By Craig Kendall

TABLE OF CONTENTS

Bonus Reports

Asperger's is not a curse -
it is just a difference,
and a difference that can
be worked around.

Chapter 1

What is Asperger's Syndrome?

ASPERGER'S: A GUIDE TO UNDERSTANDING

Welcome, and congratulations for taking your first step to understanding what Asperger's Syndrome is all about. Learning about Asperger's will help you understand how to help the loved ones in your life who have this. It is my hope that both you and your son or daughter will benefit from this knowledge of how to relate to each other.

Let's start with the basics. What is Asperger's Syndrome?

Asperger's Syndrome is a developmental disability. That means it is something you are born with, that affects the way you develop, and understand the world. Asperger's has many different traits involved in it. Primarily it affects your child's social functioning. Your child probably will prefer to play by himself instead of with others. He likely will have difficulty making friends. He won't understand social cues. The social grace and "hidden social messages" we take for granted are like a foreign language to him.

He will also likely have sensory issues, such as thinking something is too loud, that fabric is too rough, or that something is moving too fast or smells bad. These can be overwhelming to the child, but help is available, as you will soon see.

Most children with Asperger's have special interests that they talk about all the time. One child might be obsessed with train schedules. Another with World War Two history. A third with volcanoes. And so on. They are also fixated on routines and need to know when everything is happening in order not to feel completely overwhelmed.

This does not mean it is all bad. Children with Asperger's are usually very honest and are hard working when it is something they are interested in.

They are loving and intelligent in their own way. They often have excellent memories and are not afraid to think for themselves.

Are there different levels of severity?

There are many different levels of Asperger's Syndrome. Asperger's is what is called a spectrum disorder. That means that some people exhibit a lot of quite severe symptoms, while others might have only mildly exhibit a few. No two people with Asperger's are alike, and few have all of the symptoms associated with it. Asperger's is essentially a milder form of autism. It is what is called an "autism spectrum disorder," which means that it is a kind of autism, but different in that it has different symptoms and is usually not as severe, as we will see later.

Is it possible that someone would not know they have Aspergers?

It is very possible for someone to go through most of their life without even realizing that they have this. Asperger's affects someone's social functioning and they might realize that they have trouble making friends and are frequently lonely, but not have any idea why. Asperger's was only recognized as an official disorder in 1994, so a lot of doctors have not caught up to the times yet and do not know a lot about it. Since a person with Asperger's usually does well in school academically, but often has problems in every other aspect of their life, he or she often falls through the cracks. They don't get the help they need because they are intelligent with academics, and nobody realizes that they need help with other areas. They might graduate, get a job that doesn't involve working with people too much, and go through their whole lives without realizing there's a reason for all of their social and daily living issues. This is why more awareness of Asperger's is needed.

Asperger's is not considered a learning disability so much as a developmental disorder. As I said, it does not affect most kids' intellectual ability. A lot of kids with Asperger's actually have higher than normal IQs. But they might need different forms of instruction so that they understand what the teacher is saying; or need help on how to communicate with the teacher; or have behavior issues that get in the way of their learning. So in a way it is a kind of learning disability, just not in the way you would think.

Is there a cure for Aspergers?

There is no cure for Asperger's, but there is treatment. There are many different kinds of therapies that can help many of the symptoms of Asperger's. These are best if started early, and will be discussed later. Asperger's does not shorten your life. It is not degenerative; it does not get worse as time goes on. However, as the child gets older, he may have more and more difficulties simply because there are more and more advanced tasks required of us when we get older. So in that way it may seem like he or she is getting worse, when in fact it's just the challenges of life are getting harder. Proper therapy and social and life skills training can mitigate some of these effects.

Some people have questioned whether it is really an illness or just a different kind of personality. That depends entirely on your perception of things. Yes, there are some very real biochemical and physical things that are different about someone with Asperger's. They will often have trouble initiating and sustaining social contact, because they just don't "get" certain things about what they are supposed to do. They will have trouble with loud noises and crowded atmospheres. School may overwhelm them, with all the kids running about and no clear rules of what to do. The world may feel too disordered and chaotic. They will want routine and black and white rules, and to do everything the same way every time, and the world does not allow for that. They will not understand why they have so much trouble communicating with others and why others have so much trouble understanding them.

But people who have this can learn to work around all of those problems, often quite successfully. So there is hope. Whether viewed as a disorder or personality difference, it does affect those who have it quite a bit, but there is hope, and there is help. Problems can be solved for those who have Asperger's. It is not a death sentence. Some famous people have been said to have Asperger's, such as Einstein and Bill Gates. If we had no people with Asperger's, then we would be losing a very important way of thinking that has helped many people.

DIAGNOSIS

How do you test for Aspergers?

When one suspects they or a loved one may have Asperger's, the first step is to see a psychologist qualified in diagnosing this disorder. Different doctors use different methods of diagnosing. There is no blood test you can get for Asperger's. The doctor will ask a series of questions about your life history and experiences. They will sometimes give you questionnaires to fill out. They will look at your social and communication skills. There is a list of criteria that one should meet to get this diagnosis, and a professional can assess people to see if they meet enough criteria to receive the diagnosis.

Individuals with Asperger's often have high anxiety levels. These are different for everyone, but tend to be a lower grade of anxiety that is present most of or a lot of the time, rather than a sudden onset like a panic attack - although some people with Asperger's do have those too. Anxiety increases when the person is in situations that are difficult for them.

Can you "catch" Aspergers?

Someone does not suddenly "develop" Asperger's Syndrome. It is present from birth. You can't catch it, so don't worry about that. Asperger's is far more prevalent in men than woman. Boys are up to three times more likely than girls to have this disorder. No one really knows why, but some think that it is recognized more often in boys than girls. That would not account for the whole gap in genders, however. Anyone can have it, from any and all ethnic groups, all economic groups and so on. Money and a good upbringing do not preclude one from having this disorder. Good parenting doesn't have anything to do with it; you cannot cause your child to have this. Your child might be more likely to have it if there is someone in your family who has it; a genetic link has been shown.

Autism spectrum disorders, including Asperger's, are becoming more and more common these days. Once thought to be a rare disorder, now it seems like almost everyone knows someone who has it. The rate for autism in the US is now 1 in 166; that includes all pervasive development disorders, of which Asperger's is just one. Rates for Asperger's alone are harder to identify since there is so much overlap. The numbers have been growing tenfold in the last thirty years or so. Some people think this is because of toxins in our environment that cause autism and Asperger's; others think it may be just because we know a lot more about these disorders now and we are better able to diagnose them.

Asperger's was discovered and first written about in 1944 by a man named Hans Asperger. But it was not fully recognized and put into the handbook of disorders in the US until 1994. Other countries recognized it as a disorder earlier than that.

What are the signs of Aspergers?

Individuals with Aspergers are often highly intelligent but don't have a clue about anything social. Memory is highly developed in most people with Asperger's and is a special skill for them, especially when it comes to reciting facts. Individuals with Aspergers often exhibit many of the following signs:

Six Signs that May Indicate Aspergers:

1. Unusual communication style: talking in a formal, pedantic manner; or not talking at all.

2. Problems with social skills: difficulty with reciprocal communication, difficulty taking the perspective of another person; having a hard time reading people's nonverbal communication or displaying unusual nonverbal communication.

3. Lack of friends: difficulty relating to people; preferring to be alone.

4. Obsession with specific topics: seems like they are "little encyclopedias," preoccupation with reciting facts.

5. Sensory overload: getting upset when there is loud noise, too much commotion, clothes that are too scratchy or tight, or other sensory issues.

6. Motor problems: odd gait or posture; odd behaviors or mannerisms.

Can Aspergers be diagnosed in an infant?

It is hard to diagnose Asperger's in a young child. Most are not diagnosed until they are in school. You wouldn't necessarily know if your one year old child had it or not. They might be particularly fussy or difficult to bond with, but then again, a lot of babies are that have nothing wrong with them.

Why doesn't my child ever look me in the eye?

Here is something that might come up with your loved one who has Asperger's that you should know about. A lot of people with Asperger's seem to have difficulty looking people in the eye. It is physically difficult for them to do this, and hurts them to look people in the eye. They often cannot concentrate on what they are saying if they have to do this at the same time. One theory says that this is because the human face, and eyes in particular, hold so much information, and people with Asperger's are so sensitive in some ways to this information that it is overwhelming. They might not be able to correctly interpret the information, but they are aware it is there and this is overloading to them. Some have reported that it is literally a burning feeling to look into someone else's eye. Some can train themselves to do this over time and others try to do it minimally. So, if your loved one with AS is not looking at you while you talk, it doesn't mean he isn't paying attention - rather, he's focusing and taking in the information in the way he can best - by NOT looking at you!

People with Asperger's have trouble understanding intent and language. They may not communicate well, unintentionally offend people, and display inappropriate emotions. This can affect social relationships in many ways. They may lose friendships over minor disagreements and have no idea what happened. They may offend people and not know why. They may not know how to socially reciprocate. This can affect all kinds of relationships, from romantic ones, to family, to friends. They simply do not get the unwritten social rules. They cannot be social "naturally" and need someone who will take a little extra time to understand them.

Can you teach social rules to people with Aspergers?

Even if social rules are explained to them, friendship or other relationships may not come naturally. For example, it is a "social rule" that you should be friendly to people, say hi to them, and ask how they are when you run into them, if the person is someone you know. However, AS people might take this too literally and be too enthusiastic about it. The "unwritten rule" in this case is that you should say, "Hi, how are you" - but not go into too detailed of a response when the person asks how you are back, not give your life story in response to the question, and not probe into the other person's life too much. Someone with Asperger's may not know that and unintentionally turn the other person off. Sometimes simply being sincere and actually caring about how the other person is instead of asking it automatically and robotically as so many do these days is enough to unnerve the other person - since true sincerity is such a rare commodity in our world at this time! In other cases, of course, the person with AS will fail to ask "Hi, how are you" and fail to engage in the necessary small talk required by our "social rules" before jumping into another topic, and this can turn people off as well. Their abruptness can come off as uncaring when they did not intend it to be that way at all. Basically, the differences in the way they communicate their intent, feelings, and emotions can unfortunately hurt all kinds of relationships for people who do not understand how they think.

There are many variations and presentations in people with Asperger's Syndrome. No two people are like. One person might have really bad sensory issues and not be able to tolerate any kind of noise, commotion, clothing etc, but be able to communicate well when in an environment where they can focus. Another may have a lot of trouble talking to people in any situation - but very few sensory issues. Some might be able to communicate brilliantly in writing but not at all well verbally. Some might be very intelligent and do well academically but get into all kinds of fights with classmates and have trouble socially. Basically, some people have difficulty with some issues, and strengths in other areas; some are more impaired than others; it is a mish mash of symptoms. One person might have daily tantrums and meltdowns; another might have none at all. One person might have a deathly fear of talking on the phone, and another might love it. It really all depends on your child.

One example is giving speeches. I know many people with AS who are great at giving speeches, because they can prepare ahead of time, and know exactly what they are going to say. There is no interaction with the audience in most cases; they don't have to think of a response. But when you put them in a one on one conversation with another person, they will freeze up and not be able to talk at all - there is too much happening at once and not enough time to process or think of a response. So, people with AS function differently in different social situations, depending on what is demanded of them and what their particular skills or deficits are.

So, as you can see, Asperger's Syndrome is a rather complicated disorder with lots of little pieces to it and variations. People are affected in many different ways. Often, people with AS will do things in a repetitive way. This is calming to them.

Why does my child melt down if his routine is changed?

People with AS need to have a routine and need to know what is going to happen next at all times. Routine is stabilizing and essential to people with

AS; they get very anxious when they are not prepared for what will happen. Having a routine and predictability makes them feel safe. You will learn other tricks to help your loved one with Asperger's as much as possible in the following chapters. Whether you're meeting someone with AS for the first time or trying to figure out how to best help a loved one, creating a routine, using explicit, literal, verbal language to communicate, being aware of sensory issues and trying to minimize them as much as possible, and having lots of love and understanding will go a long way to helping people with Asperger's navigate the world.

Is Aspergers really a disability?

Some kids with AS will need special education when they reach school age and some will not. Some will not even know they have Asperger's until they get much older! The level of impairment differs so much for everyone; really, the definition of "disability" is something that causes you distress because it impairs the way you can function in the world. But, if you have some differences, and act or think in a different way than other people - and can accommodate these differences to still function in the world - then it doesn't really matter, does it? So, the label of "Asperger's" is only useful in as far as it defines how someone can function and meet the demands that the world, as it is currently structured, places on them. In other words - your child is your child, no matter what his label. He is still the same person he was before the diagnosis. You might have to change the way you interact with him that you hadn't expected - but he is still the same loving child he was before. Asperger's is not a curse - it is just a difference, and a difference that can be worked around.

Chapter 2

Symptoms

WHAT ARE THE TYPICAL SYMPTOMS

What are the symptoms of Aspergers?

Children with Aspergers will have challenges in many areas of their lives. Your child may have serious difficulties in the following areas:

> ➤ **Physical**

Kids with AS may have trouble holding a pencil, using utensils, tying shoes, running, kicking a ball, and riding a bike. It is not uncommon for them to be disinterested in doing a physically demanding activity for extended periods of time. Your child may have trouble in these areas, developing movements sometimes described as lazy or clumsy.

> ➤ **Sensitivities**

Kids with AS can be overly sensitive to sounds and textures. Your son may hate something like corduroy because of the way it feels. Or your daughter might go running every time you vacuum, hold her ears when a train passes several blocks away, or cringe when another kid screeches at the playground. Less common are sensitivities to smell, taste, and light. If your child becomes over stimulated by any of his senses, your child may become irritated and even develop headaches from the over stimulation.

> ➤ **Thinking**

AS children seem to think in an entirely different way. They may remember talking about something by being reminded of which shirt you were wearing and where you were standing. Your daughter may seem to pick up different facts that seem to have nothing to do with the situation. She may seem very logical and rigid. Abstract concepts may be hard for her to grasp. For example, she may not find it easy to comprehend that others are thinking different thoughts than she is at any given time. Once she has done something one way, doing it another way or figuring out another way can also be difficult. For many AS children, changes in routines or schedule are a big deal. The unexpected is not always welcomed. This is often a major problem that parents have to face. You might see this when you were planning to do one thing and you have to do something else instead and Sally gets really upset. Another issue that you may see is when you ask your son about a person and they describe everything but the person, what kind of pet they had, what color their shoes were or that they liked strawberries, instead of noticing that his name was Mr. Jones and he would be the new math teacher.

➢ Emotional Awareness

AS kids can seem unemotional at times. They may seem more concerned with what will happen to them for hurting their sister than whether or not that person is injured. Looking at a situation from another's perspective can be a challenge. Sometimes it may seem like they just don't care. Noticing other people's feelings will be a skill that varies from child to child but it is very normal for them to struggle with it. It may seem to you that they are being selfish. Often learning to think about others feelings needs to be taught to AS kids.

➢ Repetitive/ Obsessive Actions

Patterns like stripes or checks might seem overly interesting to your child. Obsessions with groups of things are common. Some common themes are space, trains, electronics and working parts. Your child may favor a certain toy for awhile naturally even having favorites. But this is a bit different. Johnny is now 13 and has 25 Buzz Lightyear toys. He knows all of the facts, has all of the books memorized and can rattle off hours of information off of the top of his head. Or Sally could have all of her Barbies lined up in a specific order, and any movement could cause her to get upset and have to fix the whole arrangement to make sure they are spaced properly. Habits like picking at skin, rocking, nail biting and scratching also fall in with repetitive behaviors.

➢ Social Issues

A child with AS will often prefers to play by themselves. When they do play they have difficulty sharing and using imagination. Often they will become upset if another child does not play with things the way they believe they should. This way of thinking permeates all of their social interactions. They seem to want to micromanage their relationships and are comfortable with people who do what they expect them to do. They usually have trouble interacting with others due to their inability to decipher facial expressions and unfamiliar terms. Most Aspies would prefer to avoid interacting with new or animated people entirely. One of the more troublesome issues for them is the inability to read peoples faces and determine their emotions and intentions.

Does the syndrome always cause serious social problems?

The bulk of the problems associated with Aspergers are social. Eye contact is a big problem for Aspies. It is something that people use to gauge a person's interest. Eye contact can be uncomfortable so their level of interest will often be misunderstood. They also tend to have a limited use of facial expressions, body language and voice tone. Kids with Aspergers often identify with the Star Trek characters Spock and Data. Both were incapable of understanding humor and are confused by figures of speech.

Sometimes though, the problem is their lack of interest in conversing with people. Often they would prefer to be alone where they understand things. Away from the confusing people who want to talk about things that hold no meaning (in their minds). They will often engage in a conversation that interests them. The goal of the conversation seems to be to teach the other person all that they know about something. But when it is the turn for the other person to say something or for them to ask the persons opinion they "check out" mentally removing themselves from the person and possibly plotting what they will teach them next. The give and take of the conversation is completely lost.

The inability to "walk in another person's shoes" gives them a disadvantage as they do not understand what people are thinking, feeling or intending to do. They usually cannot imagine how their actions will affect another person. **Not being able to judge others intentions puts**

them at risk of being bullied, tricked, or abused.

They seem to have trouble understanding that their thoughts and experiences are unique. This is a key to why they "meltdown". Sometimes they believe that you know what they need (or mean) and are withholding it from them purposefully. In play, they are not competitive but do want to control things so that they are done "the right way". You see in their mind there is only one right way and they believe the other person knows what that way is. When other people don't play by the right rules they are understood as being difficult or unfair. They also have a hard time imagining something they have not seen or experienced limiting child's play.

What behaviors might indicate Aspergers?

It is not so much what Aspergers children do that make them look different. *It's what they don't do.* You may be seeing a child with Aspergers when you have a child who has certain patterns of behavior, especially in regard to social interaction. For example, they may seem to clam up when something overloads them like too much light or too many people talking.

People with Aspergers have trouble understanding that people are separate emotional and thinking creatures and that they do not share the same feelings and knowledge because their experience is different.

Five Common Behaviors Aspergers Loved Ones May Exhibit:

1. Not looking people in the eye.

2. Throwing a fit when something changes unexpectedly.

3. Not wanting to move from one thing to another without warning.

4. Not approaching others to talk or play.

5. Not knowing when the appropriate times are for certain behaviors (i.e. acting like an animal).

How many different ways does it manifest itself?

Aspergers usually manifests itself through difficulties with language, lack of peer interactions, sensory sensitivities, lack of eye contact, delayed motor skills, communication difficulties, lack of imaginative play, negative reactions to change, and odd, repetitive habits and behaviors. Kids struggling with Aspergers may face challenges in some or all of these areas. Each area will need to be treated separately, tailored to each individual child. They have different strengths and weaknesses in each area.

Are all Aspergers children similar?

Just like no two children are a like, no two Aspergers children are alike. None. Not even twins. While they may share similar thinking patterns and affects they will be unique as a snowflake. Behaviors can range from severe to mild in every area. Some children will even seem to have no problems in certain areas. Each child will have his or her own strengths and weaknesses. Their outlook will affect how they can progress. The way they choose to think about life and the other people in it will change their future just like it does with any other child. If they take it in stride, have a good IQ, and remain teachable, the sky is the limit to their opportunities in life. That is why it is so important to help them while they are young. Their disability will be offset by their ability. The other factor is family support. Having someone to step in there and be the unintrusive comforter will make all of the difference in the world.

Nine Ways that Asperger's Syndrome Manifest Itself:

1. Difficulties with language.

2. Lack of peer interactions.

3. Sensory sensitivities.

4. Lack of eye contact.

5. Delayed motor skills.

6. Communication difficulties.

7. Lack of imaginative play.

8. Negative reactions to change.

9. Odd, repetitive habits and behaviors.

How would I know if I or someone I knew was developing it?

Aspergers is not developed so much as the difficulties become noticeable. Look over the symptoms described and ask yourself if many of those are problems for the person. Aspergers is believed to be under diagnosed. An early diagnosis is important as many habits and thinking patterns can be understood by the person and they can learn to interact with the rest of the world. One of the more noticeable cues will be paying attention to how the person sees themselves. Autistic people in general have a sort of mindblindness. They have a hard time seeing faults in themselves or understanding things from another person's point of view. They seem to assume that people know the same things they know.

Nine Signs that a Child in their Early Years May Have Aspergers:

1. Not using eye contact.

2. Not wanting to be held much.

3. Playing alone for long periods of time without seeking someone to engage.

4. Strong dislike of new people/places/situations.

5. Lack of interest in repeating or using words.

6. Not using pointing to communicate the location of something to another person.

7. Poor coordination.

8. Frequent unexplained temper tantrums.

9. Sensitivity to lights, smells or sounds.

Are symptoms in males and females the same?

The symptoms in boys and girls are not the same, resulting in the under-diagnosing of Aspergers girls. Being naturally social creatures, girls seem to be able to overcome their social problems. Also girls tend to emotionally support each other and other girls may support her, assist her, and teach her things she did not understand. Girls also tend to wish to please teachers and so are less disruptive in class so do not draw attention to themselves as readily.

They say that Aspergers is a mild form of autism. How does it differ?

Aspergers is understood as a pervasive developmental disorder (PDD). Under the umbrella if you will of PDD fall autistic disorders. Autistic disorders on this continuum are usually referred to as Severe, Moderate,

Kanner's, and Aspergers. Kanner's and Aspergers got their own names from the medical doctors that first described symptoms that were not exactly like severe autism, but obviously caused dysfunction. Asperger's disorder was not even officially classified as a separate disorder until 1994. When most people say "Autism" they are often thinking of Severe to Moderate autism. The following table shows differences between Asperger's Syndrome behaviors and Autism.

Six Differences between Asperger's Syndrome Behaviors and Autism:

1. Taking no notice of people vs. being uninterested in them at times.

2. No eye contact vs. inconsistent eye contact.

3. Retardation vs. normal-high IQ.

4. Repetitive meaningless movements vs. repetitive patterns and habits.

5. Little to no language vs. less expressive, odd language.

6. Severe sensory sensitivities vs. mild sensory sensitivities.

WHEN SYMPTOMS START SHOWING

When do the symptoms start showing?

Symptoms often start showing when a child reaches a social environment. That is often daycare, preschool or elementary school. When your child was at home they understood their environment and knew the rules. When they are sent to be with others their social inabilities begin to stand out. For children with milder symptoms it can go undetected into the middle of their elementary school years when good language, writing, motor skills and complex relationships are the expectations.

At what age does Aspergers first appear?

Aspergers symptoms are believed to appear but are often not noticed at birth. Some parents have said that their child developed fine and suddenly developed symptoms. This is not true of most cases. Some parents will notice that their baby is calmed by long periods of white noise, happy to play by themselves for long periods of time. Some do not use words as much or do not look into eyes or study faces. First children are the least likely to get suspected as babies because the mothers have nothing to compare the development to.

How would I know if my one-year old child had Aspergers?

It is very uncommon for children under the age of 5 to be diagnosed with Aspergers. Odd behaviors are often seen as quirks and a strong will. At the age of one there are limited social interactions. The following are signs that something may be amiss.

Eight Signs that a One-Year-Old May Have Aspergers:

1. Not using eye contact

2. Not wanting to be held much

3. Not watching peoples faces while they talk

4. Playing alone for long periods of time without seeking someone to engage

5. Strong dislike of new people/places/situations

6. Lack of interest in repeating or using words

7. Not using pointing to communicate the location of something to another person

8. Not using gestures

How degenerative is it, and how fast does it progress?

Aspergers is not degenerative nor does it progress. The mind works differently to begin with. They do not lose skills they already had. Situations, however, become more complex as they get older and they will need new skills to help them cope with new levels of expectation. Because they can seem to fall behind each time a new skill is expected it may seem that they are going backwards. In reality they just need to learn how one skill relates to another.

Chapter 3

Aspergers versus Autism

What is the Difference Between Asperger's and Autism?

A lot of people will ask the question, "but what is the difference, between Asperger's and autism?" Well, that is a really tricky question to answer for reasons that we will see. Is Asperger's the same as autism? If you have Asperger's, are you autistic? Well, yes and no.

Let's start by exploring the idea that Asperger's is part of what is called an autism spectrum disorder. Asperger's is a kind of autism. It has some of the same symptoms of what we might call "classic autism" and some different ones. The severity level is generally much lower. Spectrum means that there is a collection of symptoms often seen in people who have any of these disorders and some of them have them very mildly, and some of them have them very severely. There are several disorders that fall under the umbrella of "autism spectrum disorder." These include what we might call classical autism, Asperger's, Rett's Syndrome, pervasive development disorder not otherwise specified (basically, a fancy way of saying "we know you have some sort of autism spectrum condition, but we don't know which one), and other similar conditions.

Are there core characteristics in common?

All of these conditions have some core characteristics in common. All have huge impairments in social functioning and language. This can include:

- difficulty interacting with other children

- difficulty speaking

- aloofness

- using gestures instead of language

- failing to point to objects in a very young child

- failing to share social experiences

- not understanding the intent of what someone is saying

- running away when someone tries to talk to you

- not expressing feelings or emotions in a traditional way or at all

- not being able to express needs

- not being able to make friends, and so on and so forth

Most have difficulties with imaginative play, and gross and fine motor skills.

They have repetitive movements and very restricted interests; for instance, rolling a ball across the floor, over and over again, for hours; playing with a piece of string, holding it up to their eyes, rubbing it, for hours; talking about a particular kind of ships, or bugs, or World War 2, for hours.

Most have sensory issues of some sort. Things are too loud, too bright, clothes feel scratchy and uncomfortable, there are too many people, things are too chaotic, and so forth.

Most have a need for routine. Most will have meltdowns — extreme displays of emotion and distress — if they are not allowed to follow their routine.

These are characteristics that are found, in highly varying degrees, in all people with an autism spectrum disorder.

What is the difference, though, between someone with autism and someone with Asperger's?

Well, you could say that Asperger's is a higher functioning version of autism. However, you have to be careful when you do this, because the terms "high" and "low" functioning are highly variable and subjective. How do you define functioning? There is much debate in the autism community about using these labels.

Do verbal skills differentiate between Aspergers and autism?

Generally speaking, someone who is "low functioning" and more likely to be classified as "autistic" is someone who is non verbal, that is, not able to speak, and not able to do other activities, like perhaps prepare meals or pay bills or other such things that are defined as necessary to function in the community.

Someone who is "high functioning" is likely to be very verbal, and able to express themselves very well, but still have trouble understanding social rules, making friends, has some sensory issues, and so on.

But there are so many exceptions to those rules that they are hardly worth mentioning. Someone can be low functioning in one area (like verbal communication) but high functioning in another (like written communication). Someone can express themselves beautifully and clearly in writing but not be able to put two words together. Someone might need certain supports to be able to plan ahead, organize homework or life activities, make phone calls, drive, prepare dinner, all sorts of things, but be a straight A student at the local college.

How are Aspergers and high functioning autism different?

An autism spectrum disorder is a disorder marked by very high highs and very low lows in most cases — in other words — there can be huge strengths, and just as huge difficulties. Someone who seems smart in some ways might have a hard time getting people to believe and understand their problems that they need help with; someone who seems "low functioning" by our standards might have a hard time being taken seriously by people in the things that they can do well.

So, you see, a discussion of high and low functioning is fraught with problems. Professionally speaking, the ONLY difference between someone who is classified as high functioning autistic and someone who is classified as Asperger's is the HFA person had a language delay as a child (they didn't speak). Otherwise, they are the exact same thing.

But where does this leave me, you might ask? I still want to know if Asperger's and autism are different!

Well, to continue this discussion let me illustrate an example of what ONE child who is defined as classically "autistic" might be like, versus a child with the label of Asperger's.

Your child stiffened when he was a baby and you tried to pick him up. He avoided your gaze. He did not point to things he wanted to show you. He didn't talk. He ran away screaming on a regular basis. He might run into the street now, without any sense of danger that he might get hit by a car, and without any clothes on. He might smear feces on the wall. He can't talk or say his own name. You might think he is like some kind of alien from another planet - the behavior problems and complete lack of communication ability are challenging, to say the least. He might sit in the corner holding a toy car and moving it back and forth, back and forth, repetitively, for hours. Or play with a piece of string for hours. He doesn't "play" like a normal child would.

Compare this to ONE Asperger's child. Your child might have seemed normal until he went to school. Then, he started to get into fights with other kids and ask why it is that everyone hates him. As soon as he is old enough to read, he spends hours talking about the different species of trees in the Northeast—to everyone who will listen. He is often cranky and demands routine. Everything must be done the same way, every day, at the same time. If breakfast is ten minutes late or grape juice instead of orange juice, he will erupt in a fit of rage, yelling and screaming, or melt down and cry for an hour. Routine is important to him. He might not wear the clothes you lay out for him because they feel tight or scratchy to him. He gets overwhelmed easily. He seems to talk in a pedantic and formal manner, and doesn't seem to understand "give and take" in a conversation. He has a lot of trouble making friends, and unintentionally offends people by being too blunt or not seeming to understand social rules. He's intelligent, but something just seems wrong.

As you can see, there are a lot of the same issues present in both cases - sensory issues, communication problems, need for routine - but they are expressed in different ways, and the behavior problems and communication problems in classical autism tend to be far, far more severe than in Asperger's. Some people feel that autism and Asperger's are so different, they shouldn't even be considered in the same group of disorders. Other people think that there really is no distinction, that everyone has more or less the same problems to vastly varying degrees.

Almost all studies on how many people have Asperger's are done instead on how many people have an autism spectrum disorder, since they are so often interchangeable and hard to separate. The current estimate is that 1 in 166 in the US has some form of autism spectrum disorder; accurate estimates of how many of those people are diagnosed with Asperger's are not available.

TREATMENT

Treatments for Asperger's and autism have some similarities and also, of course, many differences. Again, treatment is going to be tailored to an individual's strengths and weaknesses so there is nothing that is definite in terms of "Asperger's always is treated this way, while autism is always treated this way." But here are some of the key points.

How do the therapies for Aspergers and autism differ?

Kids with Asperger's often need far less intense therapy than kids with classical autism do. They still may need a lot of it, yes, but it pales in comparison with what a lot of kids with autism need. Kids with Aspergers are most likely to need things like social skills therapy to help them understand social language, occupational therapy to help with sensory issues, and play groups to help them learn to socialize with other kids.

Kids with autism, on the other hand, often need an intense, 40 hour a week therapy called ABA, or applied behavior training. This therapy basically takes every daily living task there is for human beings, breaks them down into tiny, tiny steps, and teaches the child how to do them one by one. They are taught things like how to say hello to someone, how to carry on a conversation, how to perform other behaviors that most people take for granted. Small steps are performed and rewarded usually with some kind of treat, and these steps are performed over and over and over again until the child has mastered them.

Skills like self care, toileting, dressing, and anything else the child has difficulty in can be taught in this way.

Some have criticized this method as making autistic children seem too robotic, but others praise it greatly for giving their children a chance at life. Generally, to be done right, this takes about 40 hours per week and is very expensive and intensive. They also will work with speech therapists, occupational therapists, play therapists, and anyone else who might be able to help with their particular deficits, but the work is likely to be of a different nature than it would be for the Asperger's child.

Again, some kids need a lot of therapies and some don't need many, or even any, at all. It depends on the child. Generally, though, therapies for Asperger's children address deficits less serious and debilitating than for those kids with classical autism.

Many parents are trying alternative therapies for their kids on the autistic spectrum. Many of these therapies will overlap and benefit everyone on the spectrum, no matter how severe or mild (not all therapies help everyone, though; it is really hit or miss; but everyone has an equal chance of being helped by them).

One such therapy is the nutritional model. Many people have found that often, people on the spectrum do not tolerate certain ingredients and additives in food. Gluten and casein are the most common offenders. Many parents have put their kids on a gluten and casein free diet and have seen huge improvement in their kids' functioning and awareness of the world. Many parents also will give their kids a variety of vitamins and supplements in the hopes that these will help. Some help, and some don't, but it is something worth trying if you can afford it.

Medication is also used by a lot of parents to try to control some of the symptoms of either autism or Asperger's. One should note that there is no cure for either of these things, but certain medicines can address certain symptoms. For example, some can help with anxiety or depression; some can help with rages and temper tantrums; some can help tone down certain problematic behaviors. And, sometimes, medications do not help at all; as always, it depends on the child.

So, as you can see, there are some therapies specific to kids with specific problems, and the intensity level of the therapy will differ, but most kids on the autistic spectrum can get some value out of just about all the therapies that are available. More information about treatment for Asperger's will be discussed in later chapters.

At this point, hopefully you have a much clearer idea of the answer to the question, "What is the difference between autism and Asperger's?" You see now that, while Asperger's is definitely a kind of autism, there can be profound behavioral and social differences between the two, and that Asperger's kids are generally considered "higher functioning," i.e., more able to perform the skills necessary to survive in this world; but you have also seen that there is a lot of overlap between the two, and it is not always possible to tell the difference between someone with autism and someone with Asperger's, or define exactly what their functioning level is. It's like they say - variety makes the world go around!

Chapter 4

The Causes of Aspergers

CAUSES OF ASPERGER'S SYNDROME

What causes Asperger's syndrome?

Simply put, doctors do not yet know what causes Aspergers. Evidence suggests that the cause of Aspergers will be found in the brain. When doctors have done scans of the brain of someone with Aspergers, they have found that it does look different. The front part of the brain does not develop the same as it does in "normal" people. Several other possible causes that are being researched are: Vaccines, the Y chromosome, diet, food allergies, chemicals in products we use, over the counter and prescription drugs used by the mother while she was pregnant, and medicines used in the child's early years.

Why does it occur?

The reason for the occurrence of Asperger's is similarly unknown. Although it is believed to start in the brain, it is unknown how the brain gets affected. Various theories have yielded no definitive answers. We do know that the brain of the child with Aspergers is different, that it processes information differently and that it is easily overloaded with information it finds difficult to process. Hopefully, as research continues we will know more.

Is there any connection between vaccinations and Autism?

Autism and Vaccines remains a subject of heated debate. Most studies have concluded that among vaccinated children there is no link between autism and vaccines. However, at least one study involving unvaccinated children as a control group has found a link (the other studies only involved vaccinated persons). Some believe that the anti-bacterial chemicals (preservatives) used in some vaccines put children at risk of developing autism.

Vaccines are developed in tissues of humans and animals such as chickens, cows and monkeys. They also have chemicals added to them to prevent any bacteria from growing in them. Some preservatives used are compounds derived from mercury, aluminum, and phenol (found in anti-freeze- used as a disinfectant). However, the nation's top healthcare professionals believe these chemicals are changed in a way that they are no longer dangerous or poisonous. Yet some parents are skeptical. They look at numbers provided by the National Vaccine Information Center and the Center for Disease Control and are not convinced that such a huge spike in the number of children diagnosed with Autism and Aspergers is due to increased awareness alone. In 1982 there were 7 recommended vaccines for children up to the age of 18 and Autism and related disorders occurred in 1 out of 10,000 children. As of last year (2007) 16 vaccines were recommended and Autism and related disorders occurred in 1 out of 166 children.

Note: The author in no way intends to suggest that children should not be vaccinated according to federal and state laws. If you have concerns please speak to your doctor.

GENETICS

Is Aspergers genetic?

When you look at how common it is for families to have several children as well as adult family members, diagnosed with Aspergers or a related disorder, it seems that it is genetic. 80% of the children diagnosed with Aspergers are boys. This fact has lead researchers to study the Y chromosome for abnormalities. Although there have been some minor preliminary findings they have not yet discovered any gene responsible. It will most likely be some time before the genetic connection is understood.

Does Asperger's syndrome tend to run in families?

For reasons not yet known Aspergers does tend to run in families, markedly in males. Although Aspergers can run in families, again it is hard to determine why. Because it is not yet definitively known what causes Aspergers it is impossible to determine why one family has one effected person and others can follow it down the family line as if it were passed. Some questions will remain unanswered until more is known about how the disorder develops.

Is the cause of Aspergers more genetic or environmental?

Because environmental factors are still being studied and there is already an observed trend in families, one could assume that it is currently associated more within the family connection. 80% of children diagnosed with Aspergers are boys. Although it is believed that girls are under diagnosed, there is too great of a gap to be the only solution. Researchers are currently studying the Y chromosome. To determine a connection between Aspergers and the environment studies will have to be done on preservatives, plastics, medicine, shampoo, etc. Our bodies come into contact with massive amounts of chemicals.

How can a set of twins have 1 with Aspergers and another without?

While the chance of both twins having Aspergers is over 90%, it is really unknown why there are cases in which one twin develops Aspergers and the other does not. One possibility is that the unaffected twin is a girl. Boys are much more likely to have Aspergers. The reasons why are being researched. Sometimes one child can be affected greatly and the other has symptoms that are much milder and are often not noticed until later in life. Once research has explained to us how Aspergers develops we may be able to answer why it doesn't develop in some family members.

PREVENTION

What can you do to prevent Aspergers?

Those who are worried about the possible link between autism and vaccinations have made suggestions to wait until 2 years to vaccinate, vaccinate one at a time instead of grouping shots and asking for the insert for the injection to watch for harmful preservatives. Others say not to take any kind of medicines while you are pregnant. Still others say to keep your child away from plastic as the chemicals that leach out of it are currently under fire. Realistically there is nothing you can do to prevent it, until a definitive cause is known.

Deciding weather or not Aspergers can be prevented is something that can only be answered when more information becomes available. If Aspergers is caused by environmental factors, than sure we can work on preventing it. However, if it turns out to be something genetic, than that will be less likely.

EXPLAINING BEHAVIOR

Why can't Aspies detect subtle changes like sarcasm?

The frontal lobe of the brain affects several processes such as speech, expressive language, emotion, reaction, habits, and judgment. The imaging that has been done suggests that this area of the brain grows and develops much more slowly while other areas grow more rapidly. What you often get is a gifted student that does not know how to deal with people.

New studies that have been released over the past year have begun to explain what is not working correctly. We learn by the process of copying each other. We say things other people we know say. We eat things other people we know eat. We do things that other people we know do. We learn from them. In the brain we have neurons. Little chemical signals that control what the brain does. These ones have been labeled "mirror" neurons because they make your brain think you are actually doing what you are watching some one else do. People with Autistic spectrums do not produce these neurons when they see someone else doing things. Therefore, if they see someone making a movement with their face and they don't know what it means, they are not going to repeat the seemingly useless gesture at the right time, if at all. After a while they might stop paying attention to the movement at all.

Sarcasm is cue based. The words are the same but the voice changes. This would be considered a subtle cue and these are often missed. Analogies are not understood unless the connection is understood.

How does Aspergers affect one's ability to function?

Aspergers is sometimes referred to as high functioning autism. Children with Aspergers tend to have average to high intelligence. Aspies are usually capable of taking care of themselves. Organization and forgetfulness are two areas Aspies struggle with. **Learning management skills and understanding that the responsibility is theirs is important early in life if they are to be self sufficient people.** Social relationships can be a problem because they tend to be black and white and either over or under react to situations. People with Aspergers may find themselves more likely to be getting into an argument with a clerk because an item is marked wrong for instance. Motor skill issues will put them behind their peers early in life but will probably not make a huge difference in adult life. The same can be said for speech issues.

Why do children with Aspergers get so upset so easily?

The rigidity in the thinking and learning processes are largely to blame for Aspergers children getting upset so easily. Kids with Aspergers have trouble making the world make sense. They often have trouble figuring out what people want and how society functions. There are some things that make so little sense to them that they "meltdown" because the information cannot be processed. It is something similar to what happens when a person on psychedelic drugs has a hallucination that just boggles their mind. They break down, become scared, and lash out.

Changes in routine cause this because two things do not compute: A) I am supposed to be doing _____ right now and I am not doing it; B) I am not supposed to be doing _____ right now. New experiences usually cause fear because the child has no idea what they are supposed to do or what will happen in a new situation. New people cause anxiety because the child has no idea if this person is good or bad, if they will like them or what they will say to them.

Chapter 5

Diagnosis

How do I get a diagnosis of Asperger's?

Now that you have learned a lot about Asperger's, you are probably wondering, well, how do I figure out if I have it? If my child has it? What is the process of getting a diagnosis like? I want to know!

Well, this can be a complicated process. Not every doctor and pediatrician is familiar with the signs of Asperger's. Not everyone will agree on what they are. You may have one doctor tell you your child is too verbal to have Aspergers, and another tells you he is not verbal enough! It can unfortunately be a subjective thing.

If you suspect something is wrong with your child, the first thing you should do is take him to your primary care doctor and see if he can recommend anyone who specializes in pervasive development disorders (PDD) like Asperger's in your area. It is important to find someone with some expertise and experience in the area so they know what they are talking about and can make an accurate diagnosis.

You can also try to find this information by doing an Internet search for Asperger's practitioners, or asking any parents you might know of in the area who they saw. Or, if you have to, call several psychologists in the area and ask them if they have treated people with Aspergers.

What are the typical tests done to diagnose Aspergers?

Once you take your child to see this doctor, a few things will happen:

1. The doctor will probably ask you for a detailed family history and social and life history of your son or daughter. They will ask about social milestones like talking, pointing, making friends, what their daily routine is like, if they have any behaviors or mannerisms that seem out of place, if they seem particularly rigid to you, what their eating habits are like, if there is any history of autism in your family, etc. They may want to interview other members of the family, too, although this is most often only done when diagnosing older kids or adults with Aspergers.

2. There is no one "test" to diagnosis Asperger's. You can't do a blood test for it. However, there are some tests the doctor may do to see if your child seems like he might have this disorder.

    The doctor will look at cognitive development. A speech therapist will look at your child's language skills. A therapist will play with the child to see if the child seems to play or interact appropriately - in other words, do they know how to share their toys, do they have a sense of how to participate in interactive play, or do they just kind of sit in the corner and stare at the toys, or move them repetitively.

    A neurologist might do a neuropsychological examination, which is made up of several different things. An IQ test might be administered. Motor skills will be assessed. Basically, every area of development will be assessed, and once the doctor or team of doctors puts all of this information and results together, they will decide if the child has enough symptoms or deficits to qualify as having Asperger's, or if they think he has something else, or nothing at all.

As I said, this can be somewhat subjective, so if you don't agree with what the first person you see says, get another opinion. The amount and intensity, as well as cost, of these tests and evaluations will most likely differ depending on who you see.

Is there an "official" criteria for Aspergers?

This is the official criteria for having Asperger's, as put out by the DSMV, the Diagnostic and Statistical Manual of Mental Disorders, which is basically the "bible of mental health disorders":

A. Qualitative impairment in social interaction, as manifested by at least two of the following:

> 1) Marked impairment in the use of multiple nonverbal behaviors such as eye-to-eye gaze, facial expression, body postures, and gestures to regulate social interaction;
>
> 2) Failure to develop peer relationships appropriate to developmental level;
>
> 3) A lack of spontaneous seeking to share enjoyment, interests or achievements with other people (e.g., by a lack of showing, bringing, or pointing out objects of interest to other people);
>
> 4) Lack of social or emotional reciprocity.

B. Restricted repetitive and stereotyped patterns of behavior, interests, and activities, as manifested by at least one of the following:

> 1) Encompassing preoccupation with one or more stereotyped and restricted patterns of interest that is abnormal either in intensity or focus;
>
> 2) Apparently inflexible adherence to specific, nonfunctional routines or rituals;
>
> 3) Stereotyped and repetitive motor mannerisms (e.g., hand or finger flapping or twisting, or complex whole-body movements);
>
> 4) Persistent preoccupation with parts of objects

C. The disturbance causes clinically significant impairment in social, occupational, or other important areas of functioning.

D. There is no clinically significant general delay in language (e.g., single words used by age 2 years, communicative phrases used by age 3 years).

E. There is no clinically significant delay in cognitive development or in the development of age-appropriate self-help skills, adaptive behavior (other than social interaction), and curiosity about the environment in childhood. F. Criteria are not met for another specific Pervasive Developmental Disorder, or Schizophrenia.

To put it more in plain English, Gillberg in 1991 cited these points as the official criterion for having a diagnosis of Asperger's Syndrome. As I said, they are similar to those above, but written in a way that non-doctors can understand.

A. Severe impairment in reciprocal social interaction as manifested by at least two of the following four:

1. Inability to interact with peers.

2. Lack of desire to interact with peers.

3. Lack of appreciation of social cues.

4. Socially and emotionally inappropriate behavior.

B. All-absorbing narrow interest, as manifested by at least one of the following three:

1. Exclusion of other activities.

2. Repetitive adherence.

3. More rote than meaning.

C. Speech and language problems, as manifested by at

least three of the following five:

1. Delayed development of language.

2. Superficially perfect expressive language.

3. Formal, pedantic language.

4. Odd prosody, peculiar voice characteristics.

5. Impairment of comprehension, including misinterpretations of literal/implied meanings.

D. Non-verbal communication problems, as manifested by at least one of the following five:

1. Limited use of gestures.

2. Clumsy/gauche body language.

3. Limited facial expression.

4. Inappropriate expression.

5. Peculiar, stiff gaze.

E. Motor clumsiness, as documented by poor performance on neurodevelopmental examination.

As you can see, problems with social interactions, preoccupations with routines, and other functional living problems are what dominates in a diagnosis of Asperger's Syndrome.

When is Aspergers typically diagnosed?

Asperger's Syndrome can be diagnosed at any time during one's life. It is present from birth, but is not usually diagnosed until the child reaches school age, around six or seven. This is because the deficits that make up Asperger's become most apparent when the child tries to interact with a large number of other kids his or her own age, and tries to do a number of school related activities that may be difficult for him due to the deficits of

Asperger's. Before this, the child may have just been seen as eccentric, a little odd, maybe, but fine, or just "quirky." Once he is seen against the contrast of others his age, and asked to perform more difficult tasks, the problems become easier to see and diagnose.

Warning signs to look for include:

- not wanting to be around other kids

- playing alone all the time

- complaining that other kids hate them

- not playing appropriately with toys

- inappropriate emotional outbursts

- unusual attachment to routine and need for sameness

- lack of social reciprocation

- not seeming to know what to say or do in social situations

- lack of eye contact

- clumsiness and coordination problems

- obsessive interests

- and pedantic formal language

Up until a certain age, most kids do "parallel play," in other words, they play alongside each other instead of necessarily with each other. Once they get to the age where they are starting to play WITH each other, and your child isn't (late preschool age, perhaps age three or four, although it is different for everyone), then this could be a warning sign. Or not. Sometimes time is the best predictor, and you can never really be sure until you give it enough time to accurately measure your child's abilities

A child CAN be diagnosed with Asperger's at an earlier age, certainly; it is just not as common. If the child has deficits that are striking enough to be apparent earlier in his life, and he fits the criteria for Asperger's, a child can be diagnosed with Asperger's at any time or age.

DIAGNOSING ADULTS

Although most are diagnosed with Asperger's as kids, many do not even know they have this disorder until they are adults. Aspergers can indeed be diagnosed in adults as well as children, and in a similar way.

The person doing the diagnosis will concentrate more on the history of the adult seeking the diagnosis. He will ask questions about experiences with social experiences in life: Has it been easy or hard for you to make friends? Keep a job? Deal with workplace politics? Figure out how to pay your bills and do everyday life tasks? How do you do in crowded, noisy, busy areas? Things like that.

The doctor may ask a family member for a history of what they remember you being like as a child. You may be given a neuropsychological evaluation to test cognitive abilities, IQ, and so on. But mostly, if the clinician is experienced enough with Aspergers, they will simply observe you, your manner of speaking, your manner of interaction, and so on, and coupled with your reported history can usually come up with a diagnosis. Again, this can be subjective, and some doctors are more experienced than others in this area, so look for someone experienced.

Can someone go through life without knowing they have Aspergers?

But how, you say, can someone go all their life without knowing they have this disorder? Well, simply put, they fall through the cracks. They have just enough functional skills to get through all of life's required tasks and activities - self care tasks, school, even work for some - but fail miserably at social situations, at interacting with other people, and do not know why.

People with Asperger's are usually very intelligent people. They do well in school, and since they do well in school but have problems with social issues, no one singles them out for attention. You have to be a troublemaker or in serious academic trouble to get anyone to notice you as "needing help" in most schools.

A lot of kids with Asperger's, then, just put in their time, get their grades, and continue on in the world, not knowing why they can never seem to make friends, or seem to hold down a job, or get overwhelmed so easily by things that other people seem to have no problem with.

CASE STUDY: BEING DIAGNOSED WITH ASPERGER'S AS AN ADULT

Here is the experience of one adult diagnosed with Asperger's when she was college age. This young woman had always known that she was different from other people, but she never knew why. She always got straight A's in school and was loved by her family, but never invited anyone home from school to hang out with.

She had interests of her own, but they didn't include other people. Her interests and ways of experiencing the world seemed completely different than those of people her own age. Her family, though, thought she was just a little quirky, not too different from how they were at her age (since Aspergers has a genetic component, it often runs in families, to different degrees).

She graduated high school, got into a good college, and became really depressed trying to deal with social situations there. She saw that the way everyone else interacted and the way she interacted were completely different - but she couldn't figure out why.

She asked people she trusted, teachers, counselors, family members. Everyone told her she was normal. Meanwhile, she could carry on short, superficial conversations with people, but could never seem to sustain a friendship. She knew she acted weird; she knew people saw her as odd.

Desperate for answers, and quite by accident, she saw a TV show about autism on one night. After researching more about autism, she discovered what Asperger's Syndrome was - and realized it sounded just like her. She read all she could about it in books, articles, and on the Internet.

However, for every symptom that sounded like her, there were several more that didn't - some that seemed quite the opposite. For a year or so, she struggled with the notion in the back of her mind, wondering whether or not she had it, whether it was crazy, or could really explain the problems she had been having all her life.

47

On break from college one summer, she was referred to a psychologist who specialized in Asperger's. After talking to him for an hour about why she thought she might have it, and her doubts about why she might not (not everyone will fit all the criteria of Aspergers), the psychologist told her, "You're a textbook case of Asperger's."

She continued to see him several more times, and was given a definitive diagnosis of Asperger's by the end, which came as a big relief to this particular young woman. Now, she could explain and understand the difficulties she had had, and figure out how to work around them.

OTHER ISSUES TO CONSIDER

In the end, diagnosing Asperger's, like everything else about this syndrome, is a complicated puzzle. (Sometimes, however, you get lucky, and it is clear cut and easy!) Some people might wonder, how can you tell the difference between someone who is socially awkward and intelligent, and someone with Asperger's? Because, after all, they share many of the same characteristics. When considering this question, one must consider that it is a matter of degree. Intelligence is rarely a quality that hinders a person, but social awkwardness can be.

Disorders, all disorders, are generally defined by how much they impact a person's daily functioning. If the person is just a little socially awkward, and it doesn't impact them that much, then it is probably not considered a disorder.

If they are very socially awkward - well, then, you have to look to see if they have some of the other traits associated with Asperger's. Do they have sensory issues? Do they have executive function, i.e., planning and organizing, issues? Do they have any motor or coordination issues? Do they truly have trouble knowing how to even initiate a conversation, or do they know how but just find it difficult? One has to look at the list of criteria that go with Asperger's, and decide if this person truly meets these criteria, or doesn't. It can be a hard question sometimes. There can definitely be a gray area between someone with very mild Asperger's and someone with just a few traits but perhaps not enough to qualify for a diagnosis.

As far as the difference in diagnosing high functioning autism and

Asperger's goes, the only difference is that there was a speech delay for those with high functioning autism, and not for those with Aspergers. Otherwise, they are virtually the same thing.

Is it common to have other conditions too?

Another problem to consider with diagnosing Asperger's is that there are many conditions that can overlap with it. Many people will try to self diagnose their Asperger's - that is, decide that they have it after reading about it on the Internet or somewhere else - and that can be problematic sometimes if they are doing so without all of the right information.

People can think they have Asperger's when they might really have something else. Some conditions that can overlap or be mistaken for Asperger's are things like social anxiety disorder, general anxiety disorder, attention deficit disorder, obsessive compulsive disorder, symptoms that result from a traumatic experience (post traumatic stress syndrome), and so on.

Some highly gifted children, as mentioned before, might show symptoms that seem like Asperger's, but aren't. All of these conditions require highly different treatment and attention, so it is important to see a qualified professional who can make the appropriate diagnosis.

Seven Conditions that Can Be Mistaken for Aspergers:

1. Social anxiety disorder/Social phobia

2. General anxiety disorder

3. Attention deficit disorder (ADD)

4. Attention deficit hyperactivity disorder (ADHD)

5. Obsessive compulsive disorder (OCD)

6. Oppositional defiant disorder (ODD)

7. Post traumatic stress syndrome (symptoms that result from a traumatic experience)

Some adults don't have the money for a proper diagnosis, however, and just want the satisfaction and emotional fulfillment that comes with knowing there is a reason for their problems.

If they are reasonably sure that the label of Asperger's fits them, and this gives them emotional satisfaction - and they do not plan to seek treatment or need the diagnosis for any work or school related reason - then there is nothing wrong with self diagnosis and no reason to seek a professional opinion. Just knowing there is a reason for the difficulties you have experienced can be an enormous relief for many adults, whether or not a professional verifies it.

So, when it all comes down to it, as you can see, the diagnosis of Asperger's Syndrome can be a very tricky thing! But it is a challenge definitely worth it in the end. Once you have properly identified your child's unique strengths and difficulties, and you know the label that best fits him, whatever that may be, you can start getting him the help and support he needs, so he and you both will be well on the road to a happy and productive life.

Chapter 6

Treating Asperger's Syndrome

What can be done to treat Asperger's?

So, you have come this far in learning about Asperger's, but you still have one (or more) burning questions on your mind. How do you treat this thing? Can you treat this thing? What are the current options in treating it? Well, have no fear, in this chapter we will explore all of the current options there now exist in treating every aspect of Asperger's Syndrome.

Can Asperger's Syndrome be cured?

First of all, you should know that while there is treatment to help some of the symptoms of Asperger's Syndrome, there is no cure for it. Asperger's is not curable. If you have it, you have it. There will likely never be a cure for it, because it has to do with the very genes you were born with.

As a side note, some scientists are working on a prenatal screening that would screen for babies with autism or Asperger's and allow the parent the option to abort the baby. This would, in effect, "cure it," but has raised an uproar for some in the autism community who feel it would be like eradicating a whole population of people who, despite their many difficulties, have some unique strengths to offer the world. Imagine what the world would be like without Albert Einstein or Bill Gates, for example - quirky, intelligent people who think outside the box. Others, of course, seeing the many challenges of Asperger's, are all for such a thing. It is not likely to happen any time soon, however, and so remains just an idea. There is no cure or any plans for any cure for any living person who has Asperger's.

Do the symptoms of Aspergers lessen with age?

It should also be known, though, that as the person with Asperger's grows older, some of the symptoms may likely abate on their own; they will find new ways to cope with the world; they will find a place where they fit in where their strengths are recognized and appreciated. So how a child with Asperger's interacts with the world is not necessarily how the same adult with Asperger's will interact with the world. This is, of course, different for everybody.

Can Aspergers be prevented?

Asperger's is not preventable. It is largely thought to be caused by genes. Therefore, there is nothing you did that caused it. Most likely, but not in all cases, if you look hard enough in your family history, you will find other people in your family with similar, but less pronounced, traits! It is something you are born with. The symptoms might not show up clearly until a child is older, but it cannot just start happening when a child is older or an adult; it is something you either have when you are born or not.

There are some people who believe that the mercury preservatives in vaccines can cause autism and Asperger's. There is no real clear scientific evidence either way on this question, but it is generally believed that autism is caused by genetics. The official government view is that vaccines do not cause autism, but many parents have taken issue with that statement. This is something that one would have to decide for themselves, if they think it has any merit or not; but, in general, the most popular belief is that autism is caused by genetics.

In the future, when more is known about Aspergers there might be prevention in a sense. If some cases are found to be caused by environmental factors, then things could be changed. If it is caused by food allergies, then these children could go on a special diet. If it is caused by vaccines, they could be reformulated. However, if it is caused by genetics, management may be more likely. A miracle drug that reverses the damage and causes the centers of the brain to grow properly could also be in the future. However, much more research will need to be done to determine a cause before we can talk about any cure for Aspergers.

TREATMENTS

Treatments for Asperger's have been discussed briefly in previous chapters and will be explored in more depth here. Basically, Aspergers is treated by training the child how the world outside of their mind works. Because they have trouble recognizing that other people are having different thoughts than them, they have to be taught this. Once they have learned that, they can be trained to respond to other people in a way that will help them get what they need. Then they will be taught about relationships and the give and take of conversations and friendships. Because there are many social rules that human beings abide by, years of this type of learning is needed. They will learn to recognize social cues, body language, emotions, figures of speech, and what their own body is telling them. Physical interventions will help them get over clumsiness. Speech problems can be addressed. There are a great many current treatments that are used by various therapists -- some more common than others.

12 Categories of Treatments for Asperger's Syndrome

1. Occupational therapy may help with writing and drawing.

2. Physical therapy to help them with physical issues like clumsiness, balance and stiffness.

3. Behavior Modification therapies can include but are not limited to...

   o Positive Behavior Support

   o Applied Behavior Analysis

   o Preventative Classroom Management

   o Pro-social Behavior

   o Moral Education

   o Play Therapy

   o Assertive Discipline

   o Reality Therapy

   o Aggression Replacement Training

4. Social issues are addressed by Social Problem Solving Social Stories, and Social Skills Training which teach children social

skills through lessons and role play.

5. Family Therapy is recommended to assist the formation of good family relationships and interactions.

6. Sensory Integration Therapy can be helpful for children with bothersome sensitivities.

7. Effective Communication Models or Communication Therapy help the child with verbal communication skills.

8. Picture Exchange Communication Systems is a treatment that allows children to communicate with pictures.

9. Speech Therapy can help children with odd speech.

10. Dietary Modifications may be tried to eliminate the possibility that the child is responding to a food allergy or nutrient imbalance.

11. Supplements can be tried as recent research has found a possible link to supplements and behavior improvements.

12. Serious negative behaviors are sometimes managed by medications such as Antidepressants, Benzodiazepines, Antipsychotics and Stimulants.

What are the preferred treatment options?

Behavioral Modification, social stories or other social skills therapies and medications (when needed) are accepted as the most effective treatments.

All in all, there are many current treatments for Aspergers. Some of these treatments are less than obvious and we will discuss them in more details.

➤ Occupational therapy

Occupational therapy helps a person learn to cope with their specific difficulties in a way that works best for them. They work a lot with kids and adults with Aspergers. One area that kids with Aspergers have many problems with is sensory issues. Things are too loud, too bright, too chaotic, clothes are too tight, etc. Occupational therapists can do different forms of sensory integration therapy to help the child with these issues.

When we say that kids with Aspergers have sensory issues, we mean that they have trouble processing sensory information. All around us, every day, we receive tons of sensory information. People with a normal system will tune out most of the things they do not need to be aware of at any given time. People with sensory issues, though, cannot process or filter out ANYTHING. Everything is too loud, too bright, too tight, too distracting, their nervous system reacts over and over again to all of the sensory stimuli in their environment. There are some techniques a therapist can use to help kids better modulate sensory information that they are receiving.

➤ Auditory integration therapy

For example, if the child has overly sensitive hearing, one thing the therapist can do is called auditory integration therapy. This basically involves having the child listen to specially prepared tapes of different tones and frequencies, and special kinds of music that can actually change the way the brain processes auditory information. This will make the child less over stimulated by loud noises and such. Headphones are used for this, and usually around twenty or so (the number can vary) half-hour sessions are required before any improvement can be seen. This does not work for everyone, but has been shown to help many.

➢ Wilbarger Deep Pressure technique

Another thing that can help kids who are sensitive to touch, or have problems with the feeling of clothing, is something called the Wilbarger Deep Pressure technique. Basically, the child's skin is brushed in a certain way with a certain type of brush. This helps stimulate certain nerves and receptors in the body and brain and, over time, can make the child more tolerant to the feeling of certain fabrics and more tolerant of things touching him or her. It also helps the child mentally organize himself, and improves mind-body communication. Since many children with Aspergers crave deep pressure, this can help them relax. Generally, this is done every couple of hours for a certain time period, by someone who is trained in the method (most occupational therapists who work with kids on the autistic spectrum are).

There are many other things, often referred to as a "sensory diet," that can help kids with sensory issues. Simply put, some kids are under receptive to sensory information, and need to engage in activities like spinning, balancing, running, rolling on a ball and so on to get themselves going and start "feeling okay." Others are too sensitive to this information and there are activities that can help re-engineer the brain so that they can process it better. Often something that looks like play can actually be changing the way a child's brain works.

➢ Speech therapy

Speech therapy is more than just speech therapy. Many kids with Aspergers have problems with understanding language, and using language, and understanding the intent and practical message of what someone is saying; and speech therapy can help with this. In other words, it's not physically saying the words that kids with Aspergers have problems with, it's understanding the meaning behind the words. Kids with Aspergers often have problems with understanding jokes, kidding, hidden messages, anything that is not extremely literal and explicit. Even very verbal kids can benefit from speech therapy in that they will better be able to understand the *meaning* of words. It is also common for Aspergers kids to have trouble with things like tone of voice and understanding nonverbal language, and speech therapy can help with that, too.

It is often said that 80% of the way we communicate is done with our bodies and not our words - no wonder our Asperger's kids have so much trouble figuring out what we're saying! They look at our face and it seems blank to them - they can't figure out the messages that we are trying to convey to them that seems so obvious. Kids with Aspergers can be taught to recognize emotions and nonverbal cues on people's faces, though, by using pictures and explicitly taught practical experience.

> ## Play therapy and social skills therapy

Play therapy and social skills therapy kind of go together. Both are venues where kids are explicitly taught social experiences, and how to interact with others. Through working with other kids who have similar problems or one-on-one with a therapist, kids learn how to do things like share, have reciprocal conversations with others, show interest in what others are doing and feeling, and share experiences with others. Depending on age level, skills like making eye contact, greeting others, taking turns in conversations, figuring out how long to talk, and so on are practiced until mastered or improved. Role playing is used. Kids can then take the skills they learn in the group and hopefully generalize them to outside social situations. Group Therapy can also allow kids to practice by making use of role playing social interactions.

Carol Grey's Social Stories, Social Articles and Thinking Stories are one of the best and most widely accepted social skills models (www.thegraycenter.org). Her Social stories are stories of actual social events; for example, going to the gas station to get a soda pop. The interactions and reactions will be told and verbal and non-verbal cues are explained. This way the child is able to recognize similar situations when they happen and will know how to respond.

The degree of social impact on a person with Aspergers varies. Some children learn social skills easier than others. Your Aspergers loved one also has to understand why social skills are important to them. Children with Aspergers can often be described by others as uncaring, unemotional, rude or unempathetic. Often it is not that the child does not care but rather that they have missed something. Often there is a misunderstanding about what is going on or how they are supposed to react to the situation. Things that others seem to naturally understand about the world and relationships and communication are lessons that the Aspergers child must study and learn. People with Aspergers often do not know what is important or what is expected in social interactions. These concepts, often picked up by subtle cues, have as much meaning as words. Your Aspergers child does not instinctively know that a non-verbal gesture (such as pointing) is a method of communicating. Often they do not follow an instruction because they did not understand what was required of them or why. Learning how to respond to people and situations is imperative for them to be able to function as a part of society. Social skills treatments that teach them what to do by mapping out the situation have had great success and are highly recommended.

➤ Psychotherapy

Psychotherapy is not always used or useful, but can be helpful to both kids and adults in processing their feelings about being different. It can be very difficult to be young, in school, trying to make friends, fail miserably, and have no idea why. "Asperger's" can be an abstract concept for some kids to grasp, and all they really know is that they are different; but they don't want to be different. It hurts to be different. A psychotherapist can help the child, adolescent or adult try to come to terms with these feelings and try to accept himself as he is. Self esteem is important for kids to have and this can help with that.

Different kids will have different therapy needs; teenagers will be much more likely to need and benefit from this type of therapy than younger kids, as their awareness of their different way of being becomes greater the older they get. Teenagers are at risk of developing depression once this awareness sets in, and therapy can be a good way to try to prevent this from happening. Different therapists have different capabilities and personalities, though, and it is important to find one that seems to work well with your child.

What are alternative therapies for Aspergers?

We have just chatted about some of the most commonly used treatments and therapies for kids and adults with Asperger's. There are also a number of alternative treatments that are used.

> ## Nutritional therapy

One is nutritional therapy. This is the theory that what a person eats makes a huge difference on how their brain works, their behavior, and how they function as a person. Many parents put their kids on a diet free of things like gluten and casein. They say that their kids are able to focus much better, interact much better, and have far fewer behavioral problems. Many parents swear by it. It does not work for everyone, though. Others use nutritional supplements and a variety of vitamins. Omega 3s are one popular supplement said to stabilize the mood and behavior of some kids. One can research this on the Internet and decide for themselves what to try. Most of these things are available at your local health food store.

Many kids react to foods with sugar, artificial ingredients or food dyes, and preservatives in them, so many parents will try to keep their kids on a diet free of these things.

> ## Hyperbaric oxygen chamber therapy

Other alternative therapies include things like hyperbaric oxygen chamber therapy, where a child is put in a room with a very pure, high percentage of oxygen. The theory is this increases oxygen tissue concentration and increases brain and body function. Some people have seen results from chiropractic treatments. Some chiropractors are trained in ways to do adjustments on autistic patients that increase brain and body alignment and function.

Finally, the local school system is required by law to help any child with a disability, including Asperger's, receive a free and appropriate education. This means that they will likely provide aides, certain accommodations, and special ways of teaching for your child so they can better navigate the social, sensory, and academic problems they will likely encounter when they get to school. This will be discussed in more detail in a later chapter.

PARENTAL INVOLVEMENT

Of course, all the therapies in the world probably won't do much good if the parent is not invested in helping their child with Asperger's learn to cope with the world. There are certain things parents can do to help their child's behaviors, anxieties, and functioning.

What are some things a parent can do to help?

The most important thing is to be consistent. Kids with Asperger's thrive on routine. Everything needs to be done at the same time, in the same way, every day, as much as possible, to give the child a sense of safety and security. When you talk to your child with Aspergers, you should use a calm and even tone of voice, and use explicit language that says exactly what you mean. Do not make requests too complicated or ask a child to do things with too many steps at once. Try to keep your language as literal as possible. Try to be very verbal. If your child does something right, praise them for it. If they do something you do not like, calmly tell them why their behavior is not appropriate, and explain what you would like them to do instead. Try not to get too emotional while doing this. Often, if a parent gets angry, their anger will be so overwhelming that the child will not hear a single thing you are saying while you are angry, and therefore will not learn from the experience! They will just learn that something they did was bad, they don't know what, they're too scared to ask, and stay away from Daddy when he's like that!

What can I do when my child has a meltdown?

Kids with Aspergers are very prone to meltdowns, something that can be very frustrating to parents. These are emotional outbursts or tantrums that happen when a child is overwhelmed. They can take the form of crying and screaming, or even violence like kicking something or lashing out at someone.

The most important thing to remember when dealing with these situations is to try to figure out what caused them. Your child is not doing this to intentionally annoy you; he is doing it because he has reached his limit of tolerance in whatever he is dealing with. Maybe the music is too loud, there are too many people trying to talk to him at once, he had a bad day at school, he's worried about something, his clothes are bothering him, so on, and so forth. Once you figure out what the problem is, you can try to remove it (if it's a sensory stimulus) or otherwise try to figure out how to improve it. Maybe something has changed about his usual routine; reassure him of the routine for the rest of the day and that the routine will not change the next day, if that is the case.

If it's something simple like loud music, simply remove the child from the situation to somewhere quiet where they can calm down.

Try to empathize with your child. Say something like, "Boy, that music sure was loud, wasn't it?" In this way, you are voicing the feelings that they are not able to, and this can be a relief to them. The more overwhelmed you are, the harder it is to communicate, and the harder it is to communicate, the more isolated you feel, thus increasing the cycle of bad feelings. Tell them you love them. Hug them, if they are okay with hugs. Just give them time and space to calm down.

If you cannot figure out what is causing the meltdown, remove them from the situation if it is outside the house to a calm and quiet place. If in the house, try to engage them in some kind of calming activity, or try to redirect their attention to something else.

Most importantly, though, if you are able to, just wait it out and let them express their emotions if they are doing so safely. It is a stressful world that our Aspergers children live in, and sometimes they just need a release valve.

Should I try to stop the excessive behaviors?

Many parents wonder if they should try to stop obsessive behaviors in their kids. Sometimes, for example, a child will talk about dinosaurs endlessly, or play with a toy truck over and over again, or play with objects in an obsessive way. The answer is yes and no. Generally, as I said, kids need a release valve and a way to release stress, and these kind of stimulatory activities are how they do it. If they are interested in dinosaurs or World War II or any other subject, and talk about it endlessly, be glad they are interested in something and hope it translates into a career some day.

On the other hand, you do want to try to make sure the child can engage in some appropriate conversation not related to dinosaurs, and that your child is engaged in the world beyond endlessly playing with a toy truck, so use your judgment. Let your child engage in these activities sometimes, even a lot of the time, but not all of the time. Or let your kids engage in their special interests or obsessional activities after they have completed chores they need to do or homework, to make sure they are able to do these activities. Basically, once a child has had a full day of school, and are using all of their mental faculties to survive there, when they come home they should be allowed to relax a little, and if these things are the way they relax, then so be it.

MEDICATION

There is no one medication that can cure or even uniformly help Asperger's. There is no one medication that works for everyone. What you can do is treat the symptoms one by one. This is very much a hit and miss process, unfortunately. Different medications will work for different people. Sometimes you might have to try a dozen different medications before you find one that will help the symptom you are trying to alleviate without too many side effects. It can be a frustrating process. Not everyone with Aspergers takes medications. It helps some, but does not help others at all.

What are some of the common medications prescribed?

These are the most common medications that people with Asperger's will take.

o   Anti-anxiety medications: like lorazapam, Valium, etc. These can reduce the often disabling anxiety that is seen in many people with Aspergers.

o   Antidepressants. Many people with Aspergers suffer from depression and from obsessive thoughts and behavior. Some antidepressants, like Prozac and Zoloft, can help with this.

o   For hyperactivity, inattention, and impulsivity, stimulant type medications are often prescribed; for attention deficit disorder, drubs such as Ritalin are sometimes used.

o   For aggression and violent behavior, as well as frequent tantrums and rages, very small doses of antipsychotics like Risperdal can be used.

All of these medications have side effects, some of which can be quite serious. They differ so widely by the medication that it would be impossible to list them all. Some will make your child sleepy, hyper, manic, lethargic, make their heart race, give them anxiety, cause weight gain, make them unable to focus and out of it, give them physical side effects, the list goes on and on. But not all kids will have all side effects. The best thing to do is to work closely with your child's doctor to make sure you are choosing the best drug for your child, if that is the route you to decide on, and to closely monitor any side effects that may occur. Again, it is NOT always necessary to medicate kids with Aspergers; many do just fine without any medications. Occasionally, long term use of some drugs can give permanent side effects, and this is another thing to watch out for and monitor when considering use of a psychotropic drug for your child. This happens relatively rarely, though.

There are no surgical interventions for Asperger's. As stated before, parents can and often do try natural remedies for their children. Homeopathic remedies are popular. These are highly diluted substances that are said to help with many health problems. There are natural vitamins, herbs, and homeopathic remedies that can help a child relax, focus more, fall asleep, and so on. Some parents use melatonin to help their kids sleep. As mentioned before, many parents will use diet to help a child's behavior and functioning.

There is no one answer to the medication question. It is highly individualized, and only you and your doctor can figure out what might work best for your child, and if medication is a risk you want to take. Again, not all children with Aspergers need to be on medications - many will even do better without them - but for some, it can help!

Are therapies for Aspergers and autism similar?

Therapies for Asperger's and autism, as discussed more thoroughly in an earlier chapter, often overlap. However, therapies for classical autism tend to be far more intense, time consuming and involve intense behavioral training, whereas therapies for Aspergers involve more social skills therapy. Asperger's is part of the autistic spectrum, which means it is a kind of autism, but is generally considered to be a higher functioning kind with different strengths and weaknesses than those with classical autism have. (There are exceptions to this rule.)

Asperger's was only recognized as a formal disorder in the United States in 1994 - only fourteen years ago. Since then, a lot of progress has been made in understanding how people with Aspergers think, feel, and act, and how to help them. Many therapies have been developed, many support services have been started, and the world is getting more understanding of and accommodating of individuals with Asperger's all the time!

People with Aspergers are finding it increasingly easy to get accommodations at work and school, for example, as more and more people realize what Asperger's is, and how to help people with it. But there is still a long way to go.

What support systems are available?

There are many support groups for both parents of kids with Aspergers, and for people with Aspergers, that can help a great deal in coping with this disorder. Local doctors and autism organizations, as well as the Internet, can provide information on how to locate these in your area. Your local school district can provide a lot of support, including early intervention for kids with autism and Aspergers. Early intervention is in many cases crucial for how the child will do later on, and most schools provide intensive services for children diagnosed with an autism spectrum disorder up to a certain age. Support systems will be discussed in much greater detail in a later chapter.

Do take heart, though, because with the proper help and treatment, most kids with Aspergers can become productive adults with Aspergers. They will often find jobs related to their interests, i.e., a kid really into computers will work in the tech industry, a kid into airplanes might become a pilot, and a child obsessed with the radio will become a DJ. Other people with Aspergers will find jobs that don't require them to interact with people too much, or don't have too much sensory stimulation that could be overloading, or otherwise work around their difficulties. Most adults with Aspergers are very dedicated, loyal, and intelligent; they know what they do well, are good at it, and are prized by employers for these qualities. They don't spend a lot of time with small talk and trying to cut corners; they get the job done. So the very qualities that can seem so problematic in Aspergers kids can turn out to be assets in adults. There is hope for children and adults with Asperger's. With a little help and understanding, they can find their place in the world.

How can we help the people to lead a full and successful life?

People with Aspergers have a better chance of leading a normal life than children with other Pervasive Developmental Disorders. They will usually be able to acquire the skills to be independent although they will always be struggling and learning from social situations. Early intervention is really the key. The earlier a child is diagnosed and treatments are put into place, the better the outcome. If children can be taught early the basics of interaction and the meaning of non-verbal communication, they will be better prepared to learn from social experiences. They must be taught that something is important in order to learn about it. Each new phase and milestone in their life will bring about more complex interactions. If the foundation for social interaction is not laid down early, than teaching social skills will become more of a troubleshooting exercise. This is not to say that people detected later are without hope. Things will just be harder.

Chapter 7

Changes As Children Get Older

Because Aspergers is caused by the way the brain works and not by a chemical imbalance that can be "fixed" with medication, your child will never "outgrow" it. What you want to think about are the issues they will face at each stage. You also have to keep in mind that it is going to look very different for each child. Each social skill or breakthrough they make will help them in the next stage. But, also keep in mind that any quirk or ongoing problem will provide specific challenges.

What age group does it affect?

It was once believed that Autism was something that happened to a kid sometime in their childhood because something terrible happened to them and they couldn't deal with it. It is now understood that a child is born with Aspergers. So, it effects every age.

Your baby might not want to look you in the eyes or stare at faces. Your toddler may have unexplainable fits. Your preschooler might hide under a chair to avoid people. Your school-ager may get a reputation as a bad kid for refusing to follow rules. Your middle-schooler might have trouble keeping friends. Your high-schooler might be explosive and obsessive. Your grown up child might have trouble keeping a job or a relationship. Every age group will be affected. That is why teaching your child social skills is so important. They need you to help them meet the challenges today so that hopefully they can grow up and lead their own lives as a part of the real world.

How do the symptoms of Aspergers change through childhood?

Childhood is a time of great learning. Your kids are learning about their families and the world. They are also learning new skills, like playing with others, academic activities and how to take care of themselves. During childhood your son or daughter will be changing and experiencing change so rapidly that they might become confused by the process. Aspergers kids will experience challenges when interacting with other people. Helping them learn methods for communicating and developing friendships will be very important. As your child gets older, relationships change and new social skills are needed. For instance sharing will become less of an issue and the ability to maintain relationships will increase. Lessons will build on each other and kids will grow and learn what it means to a part of a community.

How do Aspergers symptoms change through out the teen years?

Things will change often during the teen years. Relationships will be very different, sometimes changing from one day to the next. Hormones will effect how your teen feels and friendships they once understood will suddenly become complex. Your teen may begin to see that he does not have the deep friendships that his peers have. This might actually give him the motivation he needs to work on more complicated social skills. This will help him achieve more meaningful connections with people. To cope with these changes your teen may develop unusual coping behaviors (such as rocking and comfort objects), or have extreme reactions to situations. It is important to help them where they are and support them as you encourage them to stretch themselves.

How do Aspergers symptoms change throughout adulthood?

As your son or daughter matures and learns from trial and error, they will develop their own social style. People's reactions to saying the wrong thing will do the teaching in most social settings. Working on the job with others should become easier as they continue to develop relationships with people. Sensitivities will be overcome or avoided. Coping with Aspergers as an adult will have a lot to do with the level of interventions they received as a child. They will be more prepared for adult life if they have spent time working on social skills, cultivating relationships and dealing appropriately with crisis. Personal Growth and understanding will often lead an adult with Aspergers to live a life with meaningful relationships and a vocation.

How do Aspergers kids needs change with age?

These are just guidelines about what kind of needs and challenges are typical of each age group. Your own children are unique individuals and will grow on many levels at their own pace. Remember that while they may excel in some areas, they may fall behind in others. Celebrate each step and help your kids be the best they can be. Meet them where they are.

> ➤ **Birth-preschool**

It is still very rare for Aspergers to be caught by the age of two. If the child has no siblings and is not involved in a daycare it could take even longer. They might not be interested in other people. They often have trouble sharing as they get very attached to things they find familiar. Tantrums might be frequent, as the toddler has trouble figuring out why people don't do what they want or expect them to do.

Four Effective Steps to Help Your Pre-School Aspergers Loved One:

1. Guiding the uninterested baby to play with people they already know (like you!).

2. Working on sharing and trying new kinds of toys to help the toddler increase flexibility.

3. Changing things around the house often to help them avoid becoming rigid in their home setting.

4. Changing activities often to help make sure they don't get too frustrated with others.

> ➤ **Elementary age**

As I said before, kids go through lots of change during these years. They make friends, lose friends and remake friends many times. They learn how to do all kinds of things from reading and writing to riding a bike and swimming.

At this age a strong area of focus should be on peer to peer relationships.

Four Effective Steps to Help Your Elementary School Aspergers Loved One:

1. If group therapy is available, role playing is a good way to work on this.

2. Play dates with some parental teaching may be helpful. Here you just help your child observe emotions and reactions in their friends. This is where you say things like "Wow Sally, Jimmy looks like he is mad at you for taking his truck. Do you see how his face looks different and he is slamming the other toys around?"

3. Occasional breaks at school might help your daughter have a few moments to herself. Help might be needed at school to break the day into something she can handle. All of the activity may seem overwhelming and hard to process when activities happen one after another.

4. Your child may also have trouble with organization. Use goal sheets, labels, notes and other strategies, to build habits about keeping things organized.

> ➤ **Middle school age**

In this age group kids start developing more solid relationships. Rapidly changing relationships could be one of the largest areas of struggle. The other area that will become important at this stage is personal hygiene issues. Additionally, at this stage you can begin training your Aspergers child in organizational skills which he or she will likely need as they are likely changing classrooms throughout the day in school.

Three Effective Steps to Help Your Middle School Aspergers Loved One:

1. Again group sessions will allow kids to develop relationships with kids like them before trying their new skills on their peers.

2. Work with your child to see what motivates them to take care of themselves. This will be time well spent. If your child has no desire to care for themselves by the teen years, you could end up taking on an unhealthy caregiver type relationship.

3. Begin working on organizational skills. A calendar to special book to write down homework assignments or class schedules often works well. Explain why this is needed and encourage your middle school child to check the entries every day in the morning and evening.

> **High school age**

Teenagers will be dealing with very specific challenges. The largest will be the increasing complexity of relationships. They will also be flung into a more emotional world. They will have situations where they have done something that has upset someone and it will not be the same as when they were young. Teenagers don't drop things like that as easily. They will need to learn to problem solve when a friendship falls into crisis. They will also need to learn to recognize good friendships and warning signs for bad ones. This age is confusing for the most grounded kids. How do you expect a kid who has trouble recognizing social cues will end up feeling? Lost. Family support will be very important.

Four Effective Steps to Help Your High School Aspergers Loved One:

1. Working on verbalizing feelings.

2. Talk through things that are confusing and work on social skills to help your son or daughter dig a little deeper in their relationships.

3. This is the time to focus on organizational skills and ensuring commitments are met.

4. Time management is important. Spend extra time to ensure your high school child understand what commitments they have made and shows up on time for school, sports and other activities.

> ➤ **College age**

Social life will take on a whole new dimension in college. Greater access to drugs, alcohol, sex and cheating will create far more a dilemma than academic achievement. All of the previous work with peer relationships and recognizing healthy ones will pay off. Aspergers kids tend to do well with school.

Four Effective Steps to Help Your College Age Aspergers Loved One:

1. Being involved in campus groups and activities that mach their interests and will keep them focused on what they want to do.

2. Focus on organization and scheduling skills. This will also help your young scholar achieve success.

3. Encourage him or her to join groups where interacting with others and socialization skills can be honed.

4. Encourage your child to take courses where group assignments are required. This will allow your child to meet more people and learn how to respect the time commitments of others.

> ## Adulthood

It is impossible to say what could change here. Success, tragedy, going out on their own, becoming successful in their vocation, failing at times, marriage, children. Some losses, some gains. What you want to know is that your adult son or daughter has become self aware and that they will be willing to evaluate their relationships and troubleshoot things that don't seem to be going right. Good support and ability to work on improvement will make all of the difference in the world. Although the Aspergers adult may struggle with areas, they have just as much of a chance at making themselves as success as any other adult.

What are the warning signs that my child may have Aspergers?

Children with Aspergers will have challenges in many areas of their lives. Your child may have serious difficulties in the following areas:

> ## Physical

Kids with Aspergers may have trouble with holding a pencil, using utensils, tying shoes, running, kicking a ball, and riding a bike. It is not uncommon for them to be disinterested in doing a physically demanding activity for an extended periods of time. Your child may have trouble in these areas, developing movements sometimes described as lazy or clumsy.

> ## Sensitivities

Kids with Aspergers can be overly sensitive to sounds and textures. Your son may hate something like corduroy because of the way it feels. Or your daughter might go running every time you vacuum, hold her ears when a train passes several blocks away, or cringe when another kid screeches at the playground. Less common are sensitivities to smell, taste, and light. When any of these are an issue your child may become irritated and even develop headaches from the over stimulation.

➢ Thinking

Aspergers children seem to think in an entirely different way. They may remember talking about something by being reminded of which shirt you were wearing and where you were standing. Your daughter may seem to pick up different facts that seem to have nothing to do with the situation. She could be very logical and rigid. Abstract concepts may be hard for her to grasp, like that if she is thinking something in her mind, another person would be thinking about something else in their own mind. Once she has done something one way, doing it another way or figuring out another way can also be difficult. Changes in her routines or schedule are a big deal. The unexpected is not always welcomed. You might see this when you were supposed to go do one thing and you have to do something else instead and Sally gets really upset. Or, when you ask your son about a person and they describe everything but the person, what kind of pet they had, what color their shoes were or that they liked strawberries instead of noticing that his name was Mr. Jones and he would be the new math teacher.

➢ Emotional Awareness

Aspergers kids can seem unemotional at times. They may seem more concerned with what will happen to them for hurting their sister than whether or not that person is injured. Looking at a situation from another's perspective can be a challenge. Sometimes it may seem like they just don't care. Noticing other people's feeling will be a skill that varies from child to child but it is very normal for them to struggle with it. It may seem to you that they are being selfish. Often learning to think about others feelings needs to be taught to Aspergers kids.

➤ Repetitive/ Obsessive Actions

Patterns like stripes or checks might seem overly interesting to your child. Obsessions with groups of things are common. Some themes are space, trains, electronics and working parts. Your child may favor a certain toy for awhile naturally even having favorites. But this is a bit different. Johnny is now 13 and has 25 Buzz Lightyear toys. He knows all of the facts, has all of the books memorized and can rattle off hours of information off of the top of his head. Or Sally could have all of her Barbies lined up in a specific order, and any movement could cause her to get upset and have to fix the whole arrangement to make sure they are spaced properly. It is common for children to form habits like picking at skin, rocking, nail biting and scratching.

➤ Social Issues

A child with Aspergers will often prefers to play by themselves. When they do play they have difficulty sharing and using imagination. Often they will become upset if another child does not play with things they way they believe they should. This way of thinking permeates all of their social interactions. They seem to want to micromanage their relationships and are comfortable with people who do what they expect them to do. They usually have trouble interacting with others due to their inability to decipher facial expressions and unfamiliar terms. Most Aspies would prefer to avoid interacting with new or animated people entirely.

What should I do for the physical challenges my child faces?

Some of the first areas of challenge will be found by age of 5 when your child will most likely be having trouble with tasks such as tying their shoes, riding a bike and writing their name. Movements such as running may seem odd, like they are not putting full energy into it. They may trip or drop things easily. It may even seem like they move more slowly and have slower reactions.

Early Interventions could include exercises involving balance and coordination. Occupational Therapy at school will help them work on writing and tasks like getting the ball through the hoop for basketball. Teaching them activities that work on these movements will help greatly.

They will just require more practice and repetition as they might find it harder. Find rewards that will motivate them. When is really when it comes up. Refer to your family doctor for development guidelines.

TALKING WITH CHILDREN

How and when should I talk about Aspergers to my child?

You would not sit your 5 year old down and tell them everything he will ever need to know about being a man. You give them what they need to know and what they can handle. It is not necessary to dive into an explanation of Aspergers as soon as you find out your child has that diagnosis. A better approach would be to deal with it as questions arise. Your son may want to know why the other kids don't want to play with him and that other kids have more friends. You might tell your son that everybody has things they are good at and that just because something is harder for him doesn't make him a bad person. At some point though he might need you to tell him why. Start low key. He doesn't need a thorough medical description. He just needs to know that he thinks differently than a lot of people but that there are others who struggle with the same things. It really depends on what your child is ready to hear and when they are ready for it. Remember that you as the parent would know better than anyone else.

CHILD'S PERSPECTIVES

How does it feel to be dependent on your parents for so many things?

One interesting aspect of the Aspergers personality is mind blindness. Aspies have a hard time finding fault in their own person. It is rare for them to feel like they are dependant on others for things. It is not unusual for an Aspie to view themselves as the only rational mind in a 50 mile radius. At some point kids might start to notice that their parents seem to have to spend more time helping them with things. This kind of realization could lead to poor self esteem and depression. Showing your child ways that they can be self sufficient could lead to a greater source of accomplishment.

How do they view their experiences of making friends in school?

Again an advantage of Aspergers in this case is that the lack of social awareness can make them oblivious to the fact that people don't like them or reject them. However as they work recognizing social cues it may cause them to feel rejected. Like any other teen who feels rejected, they can become sad and depressed. A good support system is very important. It is easier for them to handle the ups and downs of trying to make friends if they know they already have people who love and like them for who they are.

DIET

How does diet affect Aspergers?

There have been many different thoughts and claims made about autism and diet. Some parents have reported that Aspergers symptoms improved with a wheat and egg free diet. Some have seen behavioral improvements just by eliminating one group, or foods such as peanut butter, chocolate, and caffeine. B6 and magnesium supplements have been beneficial. Others even found that a decrease in tryptophan (that sleepy chemical found in turkey and milk) caused autistic symptoms to worsen. You really just have to decide what is right for your kids and try it out. It might take some experimentation. Also remember that for some, nothing seems to change when they change their eating.

Chapter 8

Education for Students with Asperger's

You might be thinking now, okay, I think my kid has Aspergers. But what happens when it is time for school? How do I educate him? Is he going to need special accommodations?

The answer, of course, varies depending on the child.

What should I expect from my child's school?

The most important thing for a child with Aspergers is a structured learning environment with clear expectations, and an environment that is free of sensory distractions, like shouting, whispering kids, or a ticking clock, or other things that might bother them. They might need extra time on tests, material presented in different ways, or aides to help explain social things to them.

The class size should be as small and distraction free as possible. Teachers should be patient and be willing to see things and potential problems from the point of view of the Aspergers child.

My son is very smart. Wouldn't a traditional school work just fine?

Usually, Asperger's is not a disorder that affects someone intellectually. Typically, it does not affect their academic ability. What it does affect is their ability to succeed in a traditional school environment. So, some kids with Aspergers will get along just fine in school without any accommodations. Others will need accommodations, such as aides, quiet places to take tests, more time on tests, and so on.

What is an IEP?

When your child enters school, testing will be done to see what kind of services your child needs, if any. An IEP, or Individualized Education Plan, will be written to address your child's unique needs. The government requires that all children receive a free and appropriate education, which means that if they have special needs, they need to be accommodated by law.

If the school is not able to provide for your child's needs, there is a process by which you may be able to get the school to pay for a special school that can. There are many different therapies and accommodations that the school can provide for your Aspergers child. These are decided in the IEP meeting.

An IEP, according to the Your Little Professor.com site, has the following goals:

> "It identifies the child's disability and how it affects their involvement and progress in general education curriculum.
>
> It lists measurable academic and functional goals.
>
> It has a description of how those goals will be measured and when periodic reports and/or reassessments will be provided.
>
> It has a statement of special education services including supplementary aids that are needed to meet the goals.
>
> It has a statement of individual appropriate accommodations necessary to measure achievement (such as extra time needed to take state-mandated tests), and a projected date when services will begin.
>
> It includes what services will be necessary to help the child transition to secondary education. "

The following are services your child might be eligible for when he attends school: speech therapy, occupational therapy, special tutoring, social skills group, and potentially several other therapies, but these tend to be the most common. Perhaps a self contained classroom will be necessary. Any kind of functional aides, such as a computer to help a kid with bad handwriting, or a tape recorder so the kid can listen to the lectures later, or an aide to help explain what the teacher is saying, will be decided at this meeting.

Can I bring my therapist to the IEP meeting?

You will present your child's needs, along with anyone else you choose to bring to the IEP meeting, such as an advocate or therapist/doctor of some kind, and together you and the school district will determine what your child needs to be successful in school. A helpful website to learn more about IEP meetings is www.wrightslaw.com . IEP meetings are usually conducted once a year so adjustments can be made to your child's services as he or she changes.

NEEDS OF DIFFERENT AGE GROUPS

Kids of different ages are going to need different things from their schooling experiences.

Kids under four will be focused mostly on socialization and learning how to play with other kids; what are the rules of interacting with others; how do I function in a school environment, and so on. Kids age 5-7 will be focused on learning academic skills for the first time, such as reading and writing and some basic math. Older kids will be focused on slightly more advanced academic skills.

Kids' needs for special education may change as they get older. If material gets more complex, or class sizes get bigger, they may need help with these things. It is not uncommon for older children to need tutoring or being put in smaller classes.

What problems should I look out for as my child gets older?

As their peers mature socially, a kid with Asperger's will not be able to keep up. In other words, a kid with Asperger's may do all right socially when social activities and interaction is relatively simple, but once they get into the "who's dating who" stage of preteens and teens, they can become lost. All of a sudden all people care about is who is "cool," and who is dating who.

There is a lot of social innuendo that goes completely over their head. Typical adolescents adopt a kind of "social slang" that they tend to speak in, and kids with Asperger's will not understand this. Your Aspergers child might have had a friend that they could have talked about airplanes and rock collecting with, and hung out with, but then when they hit 12 or 13, all of a sudden said friend wants to know who your Aspie child thinks is cool, and what the latest clothes fashion is, and your Aspie child will have no idea what they are talking about - and often will get left behind in their bewilderment.

IMPORTANCE OF GAINING SOCIAL SKILLS

So it is also extremely important to realize your child's social needs, at different ages, as well as your child's academic ones. As Aspergers kids get older, they may need someone to tell them how to dress to fit in, to explain social slang, and just basically give them a primer on "how to be an American teenager," because it will not come naturally to them.

This is the age when they will most likely experience bullying, too, and they should be given support if this happens - kept away from situations where the bullying occurs if possible, and given emotional support and counseling if necessary.

As you can see, the social needs of an Aspergers child when they reach school age are among the most important to consider. Since they do not understand how to communicate with other kids in the way that comes naturally to most kids - in a sort of slang, with lots of hidden meanings, and interests that are a lot more varied and less intense than most kids with Aspergers are likely to have - they often do not make friends, even if they want to, and are often picked on and bullied. Other kids do not understand them and think they are weird. Aspergers kids can become very isolated, lonely, and depressed in a school situation.

School can be extremely bewildering to an Asperger's child from a social point. Their world is focused around their interests, their routine, their parents, perhaps, and all of a sudden they are thrust into this environment with hundreds and hundreds of other noisy, chaotic, loud ... kids?

Now, while a typical child might jump for joy at this opportunity for connection and play with others, and instinctively know what to do, the Aspergers child's reaction is "What the hell is going on here?? This is scary! This is loud! There are all these people! I don't know what to do!"

They may clumsily attempt to make social overtures to their classmates - and fail, usually over and over again, because their classmates do not know what to make of them. The rejection builds up. The child gives up trying. The child isolates himself. The child starts to see everyone else as scary and potentially harmful.

Or, in another scenario, maybe your Aspergers child is completely oblivious socially. He might be able to do 2+2 is 4 and read the Encyclopedia Britannica, but he couldn't care less when another child is around him - he just wants to read, listen to music, or pursue his own interests.

But when this Aspergers child becomes a teenager, they might all of a sudden wake up socially. They might all of a sudden realize, "Hey, these people around me? They're all friends with each other! They talk to each other! They laugh with each other! I want to do that! Wait....How do I do that??" and then they may become very depressed when they realize not only do they not have the slightest idea of what to say or how to act around kids their age, they don't even know how to express the fact that they don't know how to do this. Or to express their feelings about it. Meanwhile they are likely to be the target of bullying, from simple name calling to shoving and pushing to much worse, and not know how to handle that either.

Should I make my son's teachers aware of his social problems?

Either way, it can be very difficult for an Asperger's child to operate in the social environment of a school. If teachers are aware of problems a child is having in this area, they can try to gently give them advice and pointers about how to go about making friends, or at least act as a buffer zone, letting them share their feelings about it.

A caring teacher who takes the time to build a relationship with a scared and hurting Aspergers teen can help buffer a lot of the damage that social problems can create. They can also help raise the Aspergers teen's self esteem by doing this, therefore further buffering these problems. Additionally, if a child knows of his or her Aspergers diagnosis at the teenage age, and has been told to expect these problems and how to manage them, this can also help quite a bit - or not, depending on the child and how they react to the information that they are different.

How can I help my child succeed socially at school?

It can seem a dire situation, sometimes, but there are ways to help an Asperger's child succeed socially in school.

➤ Social Support Groups

One thing that can be done is to form social support groups in the school. In other words, take all the kids who are a little bit different and need a little help finding friends, get them together, and provide activities for them to do together. Pizza nights, board games, outside activities, and so on. Whatever seems to fit the group works. In this way, the child will have a social group that they can feel comfortable with, and practice their social skills at the same time.

➤ Interest Groups

Another way is to get the Aspergers child involved is with an interest group. There may be groups in the school or community devoted to reading, or playing musical instruments, or chess, or community service, or history, you name it, there's probably a group for it somewhere. If the Aspergers child is with other people who share his or her interests, friendships will be more likely to form, and the child will have a place where he feels like he fits in, and a sense of connection.

➤ Social Connections at School

Find out what the child's skills and strengths are, and use them. Make sure the child has some kind of social connection in school, even if it is only with other teachers. For example, maybe they want to help with copying documents and doing office work in the office; they can develop relationships with the secretaries and office staff, and have some sense of value. Or give them some kind of job in the classroom or school environment that makes them feel useful. If an older child has an interest in technology, they can help in the technology department. Someone gifted in arts can make designs for school T-shirts, posters, or advertisements. And so on. Find a way for the child to fit in the community somehow.

RESOURCES FOR TEACHERS

How can a teacher best help a kid with Aspergers learn?

Well, as I said before, make sure the teaching is very clear and concrete. Use lots of examples. Use many different methods of explaining something: visual, written, spoken, demonstrated, and so on. Hands on activities to explain a concept can work very well.

Be prepared to explain a concept many times. Know that the Aspergers child thinks very literally, and you might have to work to understand how the Aspergers child is understanding something you are saying.

Realize that an Aspergers child has many sensory issues and is easily distracted. Don't expect a child to understand something you are saying if there are people talking nearby, music playing, bright lights, are anything else that might interfere with the child's ability to focus. Try to remove the child to a calm and quiet environment if needed. If the child has a meltdown or becomes upset, it is probably because they are trying to focus on too many things at once and they are overwhelmed. Again, remove them to a calm and quiet place and giver them a chance to relax and calm down. Then, you can try again.

Know that an Aspergers child might often have trouble with things like motor skills, and handwriting can be difficult. Allow them to use a laptop to take notes.

Try to always have a schedule of what you are going to do in class. If it is an elementary school class, having the schedule for Math, Reading, Writing, Science, Recess, and Lunch posted clearly on the board can help a child orient himself and know what to expect.

Try not to have many surprises, or if you do, expect that the Aspergers child may have difficulty with them. Try to inform them ahead of time about any changes in schedule. This is harder in middle and high school when the child changes classes so much, but again, they should know their schedule and have a copy of it at all times.

Teachers of individual classes should have a certain way of conducting a class, and stick with it - consistency is key. In middle and high school, someone should help the Aspergers teen keep track of all of their classes, papers, assignments, and so on, and make sure they are not getting lost in the mix. One other possible accommodation: sometimes the Aspergers teen may be late to class because they can't deal with the busy hallways in between classes, and may hang around waiting for them to disperse before going to their next class. Be understanding of issues like this.

How should an Aspergers child be graded?

Well, this depends entirely on the Aspergers child's abilities. Most Aspergers kids, as I said, do fine academically with some added supports, and should be graded by the same academic standards of all other students. There could be some situations in which this isn't appropriate, but that's really up to the child, teacher, and parent to decide if such a situation arises.

If there is a project in which a child is being graded for some kind of social behavior, like working well in a group, their Aspergers should probably be taken into account here, and they should be graded on the academic work they produce instead of their group work. But again, this depends on the child. In some situations, it might be beneficial for the child to learn how to work with a group; in others, it might simply not be possible, and they should be allowed to be excluded from such an activity. Certainly, group work is not a method of teaching that would work well on a regular basis for an Asperger's child.

There might be some cases in which the Aspergers child is given a reduced amount of homework or modified assignments, but otherwise graded the same; this question is impossible to answer further without knowing the unique strengths and weaknesses of the particular Aspergers child.

What about bad classroom behavior?

If you have an Aspergers child in your classroom that is being disruptive on a regular basis and causing discomfort for the other students, an education session may be needed. Some time when the Aspergers child is not there, with the permission of the parents, of course, and perhaps when the child is out for a therapy session of some kind, you could gently educate in an age appropriate way on what Asperger's is, and why the student acts the way he does.

For example, if the Aspergers child is always interrupting to ask questions, or frequently has tantrums, or grabs items from other students without asking, or just generally acts in a way that doesn't make sense to the other kids - and is getting teased for this or causing some kind of unrest in the classroom - you could explain that that is just the way his brain works, and everyone's brain works differently.

You could talk about being respectful of people's differences. Say something like, "Well, Lisa has brown hair and likes cats; but Janet has blonde hair and likes dogs, see, we're all different!" A mini-education course in diversity in human beings, if you will. This is only suggested if the Aspergers child is causing some sort of problem for the class or the class is causing a problem for him; otherwise, let him blend in and just be as much as possible.

So, we see that education for a student with Asperger's, like everything else, is a wide and varied thing. Supporting a student with Aspergers socially is important, as is providing other supports. Different students will need different things. One thing is for sure, though; with the right supports, all students with Asperger's can succeed and get the most out of their educational experience.

Chapter 9

Aspergers Support Groups

Think for a minute, if you will, about what gets you through each day. Is it knowing that you have someone who understands you that you can tell your troubles to when the day is over? Is it looking forward to that friend you can shoot the breeze with when your time at the office is up? Is it the connection you feel with your friends that gives you strength, energy and support to face one more day in this hectic, fast paced world we live in?

Our sense of community and our connections to other people are a very important factor in how we live. Just knowing that other people are going through similar things, and being able to laugh it off at the end of the day, is a very powerful motivating factor.

But stop and think about the way a person with Asperger's Syndrome (AS, or sometimes just "Aspies"), experiences community. Often times a person with Aspergers cannot read the nonverbal cues that tell them they are welcome somewhere, or the subtle body language that people use to tell each other they care about one another. Oftentimes an Aspie won't be able to come up with the appropriate language, conversation topics, body language or behavior that is taken by granted for NTs (neurotypicals, or those not on the autistic spectrum) to fit into a group of people.

More often than not, no matter how much an Aspie may long to be part of a group of people and feel connected to them, they linger just outside, not being able to figure out what the magical code to being with people and actually being able to enjoy it is.

The conversations of the people around them seem like ancient Greek, and they find it in the end easier to deal with their problems alone and not seek help from people who ultimately won't understand anyway. This can get tiring after a while, though, and doesn't make the Aspie any less isolated.

As a result, Aspies are often shut out of the sense of community that so many of us take for granted. They may believe that they are destined to live a lonely life of feeling forever shut out from the social activity around them.

How, then, can we try to fix this problem? How can we give people on the autistic spectrum a sense of community, a sense of connection and break through their isolation?

The answer lies in Aspergers support groups. In this chapter, I will talk about the different kind of support groups that exist for people with Aspergers, and things to look for in a group as well as things to avoid. I will tell you how to start a group in your area if none already exists. You will discover the best local Aspergers support groups as well as online ones. In short, you will be well on your way to becoming part of the global Aspergers community!

Parents also can feel very isolated when trying to learn how to best help a loved one with Aspergers. They may have very little idea how to deal with, for example, meltdowns, rigid behavior, social problems and other difficulties that often come with Aspergers.

It can make a world of difference to meet with other parents and caregivers to exchange tips, stories, and mutual understanding. A little support goes a long way, and helps both the caregiver and the person with Aspergers! I will show you in this guide how to connect with caregiver support groups as well.

What will these groups be like? What should I look for in a group?

First, I will talk about support groups for people who have Aspergers. The idea here is that the person with Aspergers will meet other people like them; people who communicate in the same way, often have the same interests, and can connect on the same level. This is important emotionally as well as for social growth.

These groups will differ depending on the age. For young kids or teenagers, there may be more of an active therapeutic approach, where a therapist may engage the kids in different activities or help them engage in conversations with each other. This is done for the purpose of showing them how to get involved with each other socially.

For adults, support groups can vary widely. I would like to illustrate this with the following example as related to me by a good friend.

I attended for several months a support group for adults with Aspergers. The group, which had about twenty members, mostly middle aged, all with Aspergers, would meet at a local tea shop in the afternoon. One important feature of this location was that we were able to reserve the entire downstairs and control the volume of the music. This is important because people with Aspergers are very sensitive to sensory input.

There would be half an hour of free conversation between the members, and a chance to get food and eat it. Then there would be official business, and a discussion topic. Following that, people were free to leave or stay behind and talk further with each other.

I liked this format because it gave me a lot of chances to communicate with many other Aspies. I felt as if I belonged with these people. I felt at ease and able to connect in a way that I had not been able to do with anyone else in my life. It did not matter to me that these people were mostly middle aged men and I was a much younger; our neurological wiring was similar in a world filled with people wired the opposite way. This made all the difference. We spoke the same way. We thought the same way. We had many of the same experiences. This is the value of a good Aspergers support group.

I did have some experiences with Aspergers groups that were not quite as good. There was one group that took place in a noisy restaurant with a band playing - no one could hear what anyone was saying! And a few groups where all of the other members had very dissimilar interests and personalities to me. The four important components to look for in a support group for adults with Aspergers are these:

Four Questions to Ask When Looking for a Support Group for Adults with Aspergers

1. Does it take place in a place that will be comfortable from a sensory perspective?

2. Is there a good mix of genders and ages? That is not necessary for success, but it can help.

3. Do you get along with the other members?

4. Do you agree with the facilitator's style of running it and use of time? Not using eye contact

Some of these things you will just have to go to the group once to find out for yourself if they work for you. If not, you can always try another group, start one yourself, or meet members individually.

Everyone will run their groups differently, so it is important to be open to that, and be prepared to either speak up to suggest change or leave if it doesn't work for you. As a side note, I find that groups run by people with Aspergers, themselves, work much better than groups run by non Aspies, but that is not true in all cases.

For support groups for younger kids, you want to look for similar things. Are the other kids functioning on a similar level to your child? You don't really want to put your high functioning verbal child in a group with non verbal kids; there will not be enough stimulation and mutual interaction. The best way to find out if the mix will work for you and your child is to talk to the therapist or person running the group, and let them assess your child so they can make a decision about whether or not the mix will work. Barring that, of course, is to try it and see how it goes. Be prepared to seek other groups if the one you try at first does not work.

Five Questions to Ask When Looking for a Support Group for Children with Aspergers

1. At what level do the kids in the group function? How good are their communication skills?

2. Do the current kids in the group interact well? Do they tend to get along? It is important to assess whether or not your child will enjoy the interaction and get along with the other kids in the group.

3. What age are the other kids in the group? It is usually a better idea to have your child join a group with children of similar ages.

4. Does it take place in a place that will be comfortable from a sensory perspective? If your child is especially sensitive to light or sound, these are critical considerations to consider in picking a support group and evaluating the location.

5. How does the facilitator run the group? What are the techniques that he or she uses? Are you comfortable with these and will your child respond well to this type of approach? Sometimes, only time will tell.

Support Groups for Parents of Aspergers Children

Finally, we come to support groups for parents with kids on the autistic spectrum. These exist in by far the largest number. In most every town or city one can find a support group for parents of special needs kids, but groups for the affected individuals themselves are more rare.

You need to decide what you want to get out of such a group before you go.

- Do you want to focus on exchanging solutions and problem solving exclusively?

- Do you want to have the chance for a big gripe session and let go all of your woes and worries about your child?

- Do you mostly want emotional support?

- Exchange stories about family life?

- Are you into political advocacy for changing regional and national policies about autism and Aspergers?

Most groups will do some of all of these things, but some may be focused more on one than the other. The key thing is to try to figure out what the primary focus of the group you plan to attend is, and make sure that is something you are okay with.

That said, I believe there is enormous benefit to going to just about any support group for Aspergers, no matter how you are affected. Even if you don't like all the people there or how it is run, just to see other people like you, or to connect with other parents, is priceless in so many ways. I have rarely ever had a truly bad experience meeting another person with Aspergers; it is like a breath of fresh air to find someone "from the same planet as you." And parents of special needs children can usually use all the help they can get.

I'm ready! How do I find an Aspergers group?

Now that you know why you should look for a support group for Aspergers, and what you should be aware of when looking for such a group, let's talk about how you find them!

How to Find a Good Support Group

If you are looking for a group for a child, your child's therapist, special education teachers, or doctors are good resources. They will often know if such a group exists in your town.

If you are looking for a group for an adult with Aspergers, there are several resources you can try.

The Global Regional Aspergers Partnership (GRASP)

The largest organization that has groups for adults with Aspergers is called The Global Regional Aspergers Partnership (GRASP). This is based out of New York City but has around a dozen and growing groups up and down the East coast and in many other parts of the country. For a full listing of the support groups they offer, go to their website at http://www.grasp.org. Some examples of locations that have GRASP groups are Philadelphia, Denver, Chicago, Los Angeles, and many others. Their phone number is 1.888.474.7277.

The Autistic Self Advocacy Network (ASAN)

The Autistic Self Advocacy Network (ASAN) also offers many groups. Their website is located at http://www.autisticadvocacy.org/.

Local Groups

Other large groups exist in Washington, DC, Portland, Oregon, and San Francisco. The best way to find information about a local group in your area is to type into a search engine, such as Google, search terms such as "Aspergers support (my town)" and it will most likely bring up the relevant information. Or contact one of the organizations above to see if they have any information about your town.

To find a group for parents, one option is to ask local doctors and special education teachers.

Autism Society of America

Another option is to contact the Autism Society of America, located at http://www.autism-society.org/, which has chapters in hundreds of cities across America, to see if a support group exists in your town. Their phone number is 1.800.328.8476.

Another option, again, is to use a search engine to find a group, typing in a similar search line as mentioned above to find resources in your town.

What If There Isn't a Group in my Town?

If there isn't a support group for Aspergers in your town, I suggest you try to start one. There is such a need for this everywhere in America, and by tapping into this need, you could help a lot of people, including yourself.

You can place ads in the local paper advertising your desire to start a group; give ads to local pediatricians and schools; place ads on store bulletins; and just generally ask around to find out who might be interested in such a group. If there is an university in your town, you could get some education or psychology majors to help.

One of the biggest support groups for adults with Aspergers in the country, the Aspergers Adults of Greater Washington, was started by two guys who decided to put an ad in the Washington Post to see who would show up. Nearly four years later, they have a monthly attendance hovering around forty people!

It is not difficult to conduct such a meeting. All you need is a place to meet (your living room? A local park? A cafe?), maybe some food to keep people occupied, and a general idea of what you want to say and some discussion questions to get the conversation started. The rest will take care of itself.

Also, both GRASP and ASAN will provide support to people who want to start new local chapters, if you meet certain conditions.

How Do I Find Online Support Groups?

There can be amazing benefits in participating in online support groups as well as local ones. For one thing, they are a lot easier to find. If there is nothing available locally, an online group can be a wonderful support. For another, the anonymity of writing online can be freeing and easier to communicate with for some. Many people can communicate better in writing than they can in person. Many people with Aspergers who get very nervous in social situations where they have to look people in the eye and decipher body language flourish online where the only thing that matters is the words that you write, not the body language that you use to convey them in.

Additionally, when you connect to an online group, you have an amazing wealth of resources at your fingertips. You can meet people from all over the world, and learn so much from the accumulated knowledge of all the people who are participating. You can pick up tips and gain emotional support in much the same way you would do face to face.

The most popular website on the Internet for people with Aspergers is called Wrong Planet. It is located at www.wrongplanet.net . This site has several very active message boards, some geared towards kids and others towards people of all ages. People talk about their interests, rehash social situations that may not have gone so well and ask for advice about them, talk about medical problems, and ask advice about everything you can imagine. They gain support from knowing they are not alone, from knowing other people are experiencing the same things they are. A current sampling of topics on Wrong Planet at this writing are topics such as childhood fears, Aspergers resources in San Francisco, problems talking on the phone, crying in public, depression, feeling like an outcast, and whether or not tell your manager at work that you have Aspergers.

The website Yahoo has a wealth of online Aspergers support groups. Some of them are active and some of them are not. One of the most active groups on the Internet for parents with kids who have Aspergers is called Aspergers Support. To join this group, you need to go to groups.yahoo.com on your Internet browser, and sign up for a Yahoo username if you do not already have one. Once you do that, type "Aspergers Support" into the search feature, click on it, and join it. You can choose to have emails sent to your email box or read them online. Members exchange practical tips about raising autism spectrum kids on a wide variety of topics.

Another useful site that has sections for both adults with Aspergers and parents with Aspergers kids to post on is called Asperger Info, located at www.aspergerinfo.com .

There are many other groups online as well, but these three are in my opinion the most useful and active ones. Doing a search on Google or

95

Yahoo will produce a wealth of other ones. Beware, though, not every online group is created equal. You do not want to believe everything you read or hear online. Not everyone will be trustworthy. Not everyone will have your best interests in mind. Some people will be kind and helpful and others can be quite rude. You have to search around a little to find the communities that best suit you. Beware of anyone trying to sell you anything. I have encountered very few problems of this nature, though, in the communities I have mentioned above.

One final note on online support. You can find a wealth of blogs written by both people with Aspergers and by parents of kids on the autism spectrum. A blog is a website where people write about their experiences. One site that collects some of the best autism spectrum blogs on the Internet is at www.autism-hub.co.uk . One of the best parent written blogs that I like is by a woman named Susan Senator at www.susansenator.com, and one of my favorite written by an autistic spectrum person blog is Amanda Bagg's blog at http://ballastexistenz.autistics.org/ This is but a small sample of what is out there.

A Final Note

You are now ready to go out there and get some support! Whether you are a person with Aspergers or a family member looking for support, you now know exactly how to find a group that will suit your needs, and the importance of doing so! I wish you all the best in your efforts, and remember, the journey of a thousand miles begins with a single step. So go out there and change the world - or at least, change the world for yourself, and your loved one.

***

The information presented in this book is educational and should not be construed as offering diagnostic, treatment or legal advice or consultation. If professional assistance in any of these areas is needed, the services of a competent autism professional should be sought.

How to be Your Aspergers Child's Best Advocate

By Craig Kendall

What does it mean to be an advocate for your son or daughter with Asperger's? Well, simply put, it means SOMEONE has to help them with all the things they need, and all the services they are going to need to assist them with their unique issues. That someone has got to be you. There is no one else that can do it for you.

Your child with Asperger's is going to need a lot of different things than your other children, if you have them. He will probably need things like speech therapy, occupational therapy, and social skills therapy. He is most likely going to need special education services from the school district. There will be the problem of how to get these services funded. It's a lot to handle at once, and unfortunately, in most cases, there won't be anyone handing you these services on a golden platter. You are going to have to fight for them. You are going to have to become your son or daughter's best advocate, by figuring out what kind of services your child needs, and how to best get them.

NAVIGATING THE MAZE

It can be a daunting puzzle, to say the least. It can be a maze that some days you feel you will never find your way through. But this guide will give you some tips on how to find your way through this maze. You will learn the most common services kids with Asperger's need, how to find them, tips to pay for them, and ways to get what you want from your school district.

Let's start by talking about the kinds of things your child might need. There are several kinds of therapies that might help. Some you will have to fund, and some the school district is required to fund. This is a partial list of some of those therapies: speech therapy, play or social skills therapy, and occupational therapy. Also helpful can be counseling and seeing a psychiatrist for medication issues.

> ➢ **Occupational Therapy**

Occupational therapy is a kind of therapy that helps your child figure out how to function in the world. Occupational therapies look at people with a wide range of disabilities and figure out how to make practical accommodations for them to function around their limits. Occupational therapists also work a lot with sensory issues that many AS kids have. They do sensory exercises and techniques that can help with these issues.

> ➢ **Speech Therapy**

You might wonder why your AS child needs speech therapy if it seems like they can talk up a storm. Maybe it feels like they talk TOO much! But speech problems in a child with Asperger's are not likely to be how they pronounce words or physically speak, but how they understand language. How they understand what someone else means in a conversation, and how they respond to that statement. Asperger's kids tend to be very literal. They will not understand metaphors or any speech that is not extremely clear. They may hear and focus on one part of something you are saying and completely miss the rest. They do not know how to perceive tone of voice and nonverbal body language most of the time. Speech therapy can help with these issues.

How am I going to pay for all of this?

How, you say, am I going to pay for all of this? Therapy, any kind of therapy, can be expensive, and often insurance will not cover certain therapies or only cover a limited amount. There is no denying that therapy for kids with autism spectrum disorders can be extremely expensive, especially depending on how many hours a week of services you are receiving.

There are a few ways to get the most bang out of your therapy buck, though. Here are some ideas from people who have had ample experience with the insurance system. The first thing is to know your insurance coverage frontwards and backwards. Know exactly what services they cover and what they don't, how much you will have to pay out of pocket, what the deductible is, if it covers mental health and so on. And if the answers are not favorable, consider switching to an insurance plan with a more favorable coverage plan, if possible.

Another thing, suggests Lisa Jo Rudy of the About.com autism site, is to know the insurance billing codes for the therapies your child receives, and possible ways to get around them. In other words, certain codes will cost more to bill and might be able to be interchanged with other codes. You can discuss this with your child's therapist.

On a similar note, she says, you can get "creative" with the billing process for therapies. Insurance companies might put a cap on how many autism services your child can receive, but if your child is receiving occupational therapy for a physical issue related to autism, like low muscle tone, perhaps you can bill it as physical therapy instead - since that is what it really is.

Another thing to do is to research any state funded health insurance programs your state might provide to see if you can get some coverage under those.

Of course, as I said, many of these programs are covered by your local school district. We will get to that shortly. But even if you do receive some services from your school district, you may want to supplement them with private ones.

What if you still can't afford it?

If therapies for your child are still breaking the bank, consider trying to use local college students who are majoring in psychology, education or special education to help you with your Asperger's child. By researching various therapies on the Internet and using the knowledge that these students already have, you may be able to put together a home therapy program for a substantially less expensive amount. Obviously, college students cannot do everything that trained professionals can, but they can help a lot with some things, like basic social skills therapy and training, and just giving you a break when you need it.

What about respite care?

There often exist organizations in many cities and states whose main focus is to provide respite care for parents whose children have disabilities. Sometimes these are funded by the state and sometimes they are private. They have trained individuals who can watch your child for a few hours, or even a day or two, to give you a break when you really need it.

What do I need to do when my Asperger's child goes to school?

This can be by far the most complicated and difficult part of trying to help your child. But it doesn't have to be. Much has been written on this subject; the following is just a summary of some of the more important information that is out there.

Because of their various issues, kids with Asperger's often need to have aides and different kinds of special education programs when they go to school. By law, your school district is required to give every child a "free and appropriate" education. That means that if they have a disability, they are required to provide services to help the child. This is called an IEP, or an Individualized Education Plan.

The problem is that the school district and the parents will quite often disagree on what constitutes an "appropriate" education for the child. Unfortunately, the school district often is focused on the bottom line, that is, how much special education services cost them. Their goal is often to spend as little money as possible on your child while still passing it off as an appropriate, and helpful, education. This is not to say that every school district is like this, but many are. If you feel your school is not giving your child the services he needs, you will have to learn to be your child's advocate to fight for his needs.

What kind of services might your child need? Well, it depends on the individual child. Many kids need speech therapy and occupational therapy, as we have already seen. Many need an aide to help them with behavioral problems to keep them focused and calm during school. Aides can also help explain to your child confusing social situations that might come up during school hours. Many need to be placed in specialized classrooms, or have other accommodations. The professionals in your school as well as any therapists or doctors you have seen for your child can best tell you what services your child will need to be successful in school.

TEN ESSENTIALS FOR PREPARING FOR YOUR CHILD'S IEP MEETING

So the bottom line is you will have to be prepared to fight for what your child needs. Every year, at the start of the school year, an IEP meeting is scheduled with parents, teachers, and other professionals to decide what services the child needs. Many parents find these meetings quite difficult, but here are ten tips that will help you get the most out of them, and the school year that follows.

1. **First of all, come prepared**. Research therapies that you think your child would benefit from; have statistics to back you up on the efficacy of these programs for similar children; and have plenty of documentation from your child's doctors and therapists stating that they feel your child needs certain services.

2. **Make sure you stay calm, focused, and polite at all times.** This works much better if it does not become adversarial. Remember the old phrase, "You catch more bees with honey than vinegar?" Well, you want to try to make friends with the school district administrators if you can. You want them to like you so they will be more likely to give you what you want. That doesn't mean you shouldn't be firm in asking for what you want, but try to do it in a way that shows you have considered their position, but here is what you think is necessary for your child.

3. **Of course, politeness does not work at all times**. One strategy that the website Wrightslaw.com reports is the following.

   > Some administrators will consider parents "know it alls" and feel insecure by the knowledge that the parents have. In this case, you can try to ask lots of leading questions to lead the teachers and administrators into the same solution you were thinking of, but this way, they came up with it, so they may feel more comfortable with the solution!

4. **Educate yourself on the law.** There are many laws governing special education, and what services schools are required to provide to students with disabilities. Knowing these ahead of time will help you present your case better and show the school that you are serious.

5. **Consider finding an advocate to come with you.** There are certain people trained in special education law that help parents fight for the programs their kids need, and attend IEP meetings to help with this goal. They can be a great source of support.

6. **Visit the website www.wrightslaw.com** . This website is your one stop shopping site, so to speak, on everything you could possibly ever hope to know on how to get services for your Asperger's child. There is a book called "Wrightslaw: From Emotions to Advocacy," by Pam Wright and Pete Wright, that will tell you everything you need to know about becoming an effective advocate for your special needs son or daughter. A lot of the information and useful tips are provided on their website as well.

7. **Make sure you follow up with your child's teachers** to see that the agreement worked out in the IEP meeting is what is actually happening for your child. You will need to make sure he is getting the right number of hours of services, that his teachers are actually trained in the methods approved, and so on. You can always file a complaint or ask for another meeting if these things are not being done, but you will have to monitor them for yourself.

8. **Use legal recourse as a last resort.** Many parents have had to sue their school districts to get an appropriate education for their kids. This is not necessary in every case!, but it does happen, and it is helpful to know that it is an option if you can't get services in any other way. There are people that can help you with this process if needed; resources related to this are listed on the website above.

9. **Teacher meetings.** At the start of the school year, and other times as needed, meet with your child's teachers individually. Bring the IEP with you, and discuss your child's needs, to make sure you are on the same page.

10. **Keep a detailed notebook**. Many parents have suggested having a notebook that serves as a communication log to help them keep up with how their child is doing. The teacher will write about how your child is progressing or any problems he might be having, and ask any questions that he needs to ask.

If all else fails and the school district refuses to provide any services or inadequate services for your child - and you have exhausted every other option - it is possible to sue the school for placement in a private special education school, which may better meet the needs of your child. If you can prove that your public school cannot meet the needs of your child in an appropriate way, then the school will be required to pay for alternative education. This is not necessarily easy to do, but it does happen.

If you follow all of the above tips, then you will be well on your way to ensuring a successful school year for your child. Hopefully, you will be able to find a mix of private and publicly funded services that will help your child get the most out of his life and help him reach his potential.

A NOTE ABOUT ADVOCACY FOR ADULTS WITH ASPERGER'S

Advocacy does not stop when a child reaches eighteen. There are a whole slew of things that an Asperger's adult can do to advocate for him or herself. Unfortunately, there are not nearly as many services or support for adults with Asperger's as there are for kids with Asperger's. But that doesn't mean there is nothing you can do.

What if I am having trouble keeping a job?

Depending on your needs, there are different state agencies that may be able to help you. If you are having difficulty getting or keeping a job, your local Vocational Rehabilitation center can assist with this. If you are in need of counseling, there are often mental health centers where you can get this free, if you make under a certain income. If you don't have enough money for an apartment, there is something called a Section 8 voucher that can help pay for your housing. Be warned, though, that waiting lists for this can run extremely long, often even as much as one to two years. Finally, anyone with a disability severe enough that they are not able to work in any way can apply for Social Security Disability or Supplemental Security Income benefits. You may also be eligible, through the state

Developmental Disabilities department or other organizations, for a caseworker to help you manage all of this.

Test taking is stressful for me in college. What can I do?

If you are a college student, you will need to advocate for your needs at your college as well. There are usually disability centers in almost every college and university that can help you with any problems that might arise. You may be eligible for extra time on tests, taking the test in a different area with fewer distractions, peer mentors, counseling, support groups, or any other accommodations that will help you with your disability. The key is to ask, and find out what is available.

Finally, a note on a different kind of self advocacy for adults. There is an organization called ASAN - the Autistic Self Advocacy Network - whose main purpose is to help autistic spectrum adults advocate for themselves. They aim to try to show the strengths of people with Asperger's and autism in the media, and to effect political change that will help people with Asperger's and autism. They also provide social support for people with Asperger's. Their website is at http://www.autisticadvocacy.org. There is also an organization called GRASP, the Global Regional Asperger's Partnership, which has support group networks for adults with Asperger's all over the country. Their website is at www.grasp.org. Part of advocating for yourself is finding support and like minded people that will help you grow as a person and support your emotional needs.

So, as you can see, there are all kinds of different ways to advocate for yourself or your loved one who has Asperger's. From in home therapy to creating school based programs, to finding programs that will support adults with Asperger's, there are no shortage of ways to improve the quality of life for your loved one with Asperger's. So get out there and effect some change!

An Asperger's Syndrome Guide

Bonus Report

Making the Transition to Adulthood

By Craig Kendall

ADULTS AND ASPERGER'S

Well, now that you have come this far, you are probably wondering one thing. What happens in adulthood? What do I have to look forward to? What happens when my little Aspie kid gets to be college age, gets to be working age? How will they survive in the world?

This might be a topic that worries you quite a bit, and frankly, from conversations I have had with young Aspergers adults, it is sometimes a topic that worries them quite a bit, too. There are a lot of obstacles in place for someone with Asperger's to succeed in the world. But it can be done. There are some hints and shortcuts, ways to get around some of the problems that can arise in adulthood. In this report, you will learn about some of the most common obstacles for an adult with Asperger's, and ways to get around them.

Assimilating into an adult world

First, you might wonder, can my child with AS be assimilated into the adult world? Yes. You know how when they were younger, all they wanted to do was take apart toys and put them back together again? Fast forward ten years, and they have the makings to be a brilliant engineer. Your little Aspie interested in the radio can become a DJ; your non-social techno-loving computer geek son can have a brilliant career in Silicon Valley doing computer work. Many Aspies have great computer and technical skills which can be very useful in those industries.

Whatever interest an Aspie has, it can usually be translated into a career. Most Aspies - by the term Aspie we mean a person with Asperger's Syndrome - have several qualities that can make them ideal employees. They are loyal; they usually have a great work ethic; they are often very concerned about being punctual and doing a good job, and they know a lot about the topic at hand, if it is something that is an interest of theirs. They will not be likely to spend all their time at work gossiping by the water cooler; instead, they will get things done.

People with AS can be ideal employees

These qualities can make a person with AS an ideal employee; however, one has to find an employer that is willing to overlook the problems that an AS employee can present (not good at small talk or office politics, sensory issues, doesn't understand hidden rules) in order to see the gem they have and hire your AS kid in the first place. Or, they need to be coached in things like how to dress, how to make small talk, how to deal with office politics and so on in order to have a better chance of succeeding.

Some people with AS are able to fit into society quite nicely, and others have more difficulty. As with everything else, your mileage may vary. It depends on a lot of things; the adult with AS's particular strengths and weaknesses, his ability to cope with change and new things, his support system, the level of understanding people in his life have of how to deal with him, whether he can find a supportive work environment suited to him - in other words, it comes down to a combination of hard work and just plain luck. It will work for some people, even most people, but admittedly, not everyone will achieve the same level of success as everyone else.

You may have to change your definition of success

Success is a subjective word, when you get right down to it. Any parent of a child with AS is going to have to change their definition of success when they realize their child has AS. Success for some people is working a traditional 9-5 job at an office or company. For others, it might be doing some freelance writing from home. Some might start their own businesses. Some might work in the tech industry, developing software or fixing computers. Some might go to college, and some might not.

And some might have too much difficulty to hold down a traditional job, and might do volunteer work instead. Some might have to go on disability to get by, and fill their time with their interests, with support groups, therapy, or as much socialization as they can get. (Or some might not be interested in anything social at all.) Some might spend their time on various hobbies of various intensity; some might need support workers, some might not.

Most will find some degree of happiness in their life, most likely from their special interests or hobbies, whether they are able to work or not. Everyone has different degrees of what society would call "success," but there are at least some social service nets to catch those people who cannot manage to work on their own, and they can usually manage to develop a somewhat satisfying life working around their problems and focusing on their interests in these cases.

Making the transition from school

So, how will adults with Asperger's function in society? What kind of life will they lead? It is impossible to say until your AS child gets to that stage; but the important thing is to support them in whatever capabilities and abilities they do have.

When your child is getting ready to leave high school, all support workers, teachers, therapists and people who have been involved in the child's care, as well as the young adult himself and parents, should and do usually have a meeting to decide what is appropriate for the young adult to do next.

Does a four year college seem like it will work for them? A two year college? Close to home or far away? What practical issues need to be worked out before that can happen? Would a technical college work better? Or, are they just not suited to college? Can they instead get a job right out of high school? Do they need to live at home for a while and get support at home while they work? Or can they live on their own? Or, perhaps, is work not possible at the present moment? If they do live on their own, do they need support for any daily living activities, like cooking, paying bills, organizing things, transportation to appointments, knowing what to do in case of emergencies? This can vary so much, depending on the child, that it is impossible to tell until your child reaches the age where it needs to be decided.

Provide support in whatever they need

So, the best way to support them, then, is to support them in whatever they, and you, decide. To love them unconditionally and not make them feel ashamed of their limitations; to provide practical support like "How do I cook a chicken breast?" and " How do I make the smoke alarm stop beeping?" if that is what they need, emotional support for a lonely child at college if that is what they need, and so on.

Anticipate and prepare for problems

Be aware of problems that might come up in any given situation and try to prepare for them; make sure you know who your child can turn to for support at college, try to get any special accommodations needed ahead of time; try to problem solve any issues that might come up at a job with your son or daughter; and make sure your child knows what to do or who to call if any of the common problems one faces when living alone come up if that is the scenario that they choose. Above all, just be there.

It is possible, as discussed at length before, for a person to be diagnosed with AS at any age, even as an adult. Oftentimes someone will have all the symptoms and problems of AS all of their life but no one was able to put a label or name to it until they got older, so they just did the best they could with what hey had. Often a diagnosis at a later age comes as a great relief to the person being diagnosed, as it explains the reason for all their earlier difficulties, and gives them strategies for coping.

Adults with AS have more or less the same issues as children with AS; it's just that most of them have learned how to work around them better or control them better. They have the same social issues, sensory issues, and other problems; and as the demands of their lives change, they may either have more difficulty with these issues, or less, depending on their environment, the support they receive, and the individual person.

In some adults, a lot of their AS symptoms will have disappeared by the time they get to adulthood; they have either "grown out" of some of their more difficult issues, or they have learned ways to manage them. In others, the issues are the same, but with a slightly different presentation, i.e., a child who had tantrums when told to wear scratchy clothes becomes the adult who can't find a job because he or she can not tolerate wearing acceptable clothes (they just might become less vocal about it). A child with AS always becomes an adult with AS; AS doesn't just go away. The key is to find ways to work around the issues it presents. (For example, to follow the last example, find a job that allows for casual clothes.)

Now that we have talked about what the future holds for adults with Asperger's in generalities, we will now discuss the most common daily living problems that adults with Asperger's face in specific.

COMMON ISSUES FOR ADULTS WITH ASPERGER'S:

1. SOCIAL ISSUES

One of the hardest things that adults with Asperger's face is navigating their social world. They are often very lonely because there is no natural or easy way for them to form social relationships. Most people when they get older have friends from work or other interest groups. People with AS have trouble with small talk and appropriate conversation, and come off awkwardly to other people. They talk too much about their interests, forget to ask how the other person is doing, don't understand pacing in conversation, and so on. Therefore, it is hard for them to make friends with people not willing to take the time to understand them.

Dealing with Isolation, loneliness and depression

Isolation, loneliness, and depression can be very hard to deal with. Some adults with AS deal with this with therapy and support groups; others try to find friends in interest groups, such as movies or knitting or so on. Some do have success making friends from work or other activities. Some find that seeking out other people with some kind of difference or illness is helpful as these people are likely to be more understanding of differences in a person.

Dating and relationships

Dating is one of the most common complaints an adult with Asperger's has about his or her life. Dating is very difficult for adults with AS. They don't understand a lot of the social rules about dating; they don't know where to meet people; they don't know how to send off the nonverbal social cues that lets other people know they're interested. They come off too strong, and in a man, that can seem creepy; if a man seems over interested, even when he has good intentions, he can even come off as a stalker. Women also are often misunderstood. Social anxiety issues might and do often prevent both genders from pursuing a relationship once started, or initiating anything to begin with.

Not all adults with Asperger's will be interested in dating; some are not, and that is fine; but most are interested, just the same as people without Asperger's.

Workplace politics

Workplace politics are very difficult for people with Asperger's. They do not understand things that are not explicit. They do not understand hidden messages. If someone tells them to do X, Y and Z assignment by X date in X way, they are fine. But problems can arise if it is *assumed* they know how to do it, that they know they are supposed to do it, that they know when it is due BUT have not been told this explicitly. In this case, they will probably not realize they have to do it—and it won't get done.

Making small talk at social gatherings, Christmas parties, and the water cooler is difficult and might cost them "points" as they are not seen as "team players" even if they do good work. They might be hard workers but not recognized as such since they don't "grease the wheels socially."

2. SENSORY ISSUES

Sensory issues can be a major impediment for adults as well as kids in dealing with the world around them. Everything is too loud; they can't wear the appropriate clothes because the right clothes are too tight or restrictive or the tie bothers them; they cannot focus with too much going on at once, and the world is a chaotic place; they are very prone to going into a state of overload and not being able to deal with the world.

This also comes up a lot in the workplace; many people with AS cannot concentrate if there are too many people talking around them, or someone with heavy perfume, or the lights are too bright, or so on.

3. ORGANIZATION/EXECUTIVE FUNCTION ISSUES

Adults with AS can have a hard time being organized, and small details can confuse and overwhelm them. They sometimes cannot see the larger picture and get fixated on a small detail of an otherwise solvable problem.

Sometimes they have trouble figuring when things need to be done, and what steps need to be taken to do them.

Often they have trouble figuring out how to work within government systems, and doing things like paying bills.

Adults with AS do not do well with surprises and changes to their routine or environment. For example, if they are overcharged on a bill, if a bus or cab does not come on time, if something breaks, if someone is unexpectedly angry with them; if there is some other change to their routine, and they don't know how to deal with it, this can be very overwhelming and make them feel very unstable.

Support people can help the person with AS understand the change by explaining how and why it happened and what the steps necessary to resolve it are. You might say that flexibility is not a strength for those with AS, to put it mildly. Adults with AS can also be helped to deal with changes in their environment if they are warned ahead of time and have enough time to plan out what they are going to do to accommodate the change. Planning is very important to the adult with AS.

Again, this is not a blanket statement true of every person with AS; most with AS have these problems, but all to very different degrees.

There are many issues an adult with AS may face in securing employment, which is a large enough issue that it will be discussed in the next section.

EMPLOYMENT ISSUES FOR ADULTS WITH ASPERGER'S

There is a rather high unemployment or underemployment (a term that refers to those who have jobs, but are too low paying or do not suit the person's capabilities) for adults with Asperger's. It is not uncommon for someone with a master's or higher degree to be un or underemployed. There are several problems that contribute to this issue, and make the workplace a difficult place for a person with AS. Finding and keeping a job can be a difficult thing for a person with AS.

1. THE INTERVIEW

One of the biggest, if not the biggest, problems for adults with AS and employment is getting through the initial interview. Your kid with AS can be the brightest, sharpest person out there, can know the job inside out, but unless he can connect with the person doing the interview socially, and can come across well, they will never get past the front door.

People with AS do not do small talk well; might answer questions in a far too explicit manner or say nothing at all; give too much detail about their faults when it is not needed; not look people in the eye; and seem excessively nervous and fidgety, which is a sign to most interviewers that they are not prepared or right for the job - when, in fact, they are like that all the time.

People with AS can be trained in how to get through an interview, how to look people in the eye, how to answer questions the right way, but they are often going to have an air of anxiety pervading them that they can't rid of no matter how much they try, and the interviewers pick up on this and often seem them negatively for it. Not all, but a lot of them.

2. OFFICE POLITICS

As discussed earlier, people with AS do not do well reading hidden messages or understanding subtle social rules of a workplace. They might find themselves in some kind of pickle or social misunderstanding and have no idea how they got there. They might not do enough "schmoozing," or going to company Christmas parties and such, and be seen unfavorably for that, no matter how good their work is.

3. FINDING SOMETHING THAT SUITS INTERESTS AND STRENGTHS

If the work is something the person with AS is not interested in, it will be hard for them to be motivated enough to focus on. This is true for all people, of course, but can be particularly true for those with AS. On the flip side, if it is something they have an interest in, they will be extremely dedicated and loyal, and most likely far more productive than their fellow employees - they actually want to be there and enjoy the work.

4. SENSORY ISSUES IN THE WORKPLACE

This can be one of the biggest problems for people with AS in the workplace. People talking in the next cubicle, even someone chewing gum or playing with a stapler, or swinging their foot back and forth - everything can be enormously distracting and bothersome to the adult with AS.

Food and perfume smells can be hard to deal with. Bright lights, or not enough lights, uncomfortable chairs, computer screen glare, even the feel of the telephone as they are holding it - depending on their level of sensory integration difficulty, the workplace can be a very hostile and overwhelming environment indeed for the adult with AS. And, of course, jobs that demand too much social interaction from an adult with AS can be draining and almost impossible for them to deal with.

Work accommodations

Many adults with AS have found that they can work around some, but not all, of these issues by structuring their world. Ways that can help someone with AS manage a work environment can include wearing headphones to block noise, only going to places they know will not be too crowded, or asking for a separate office at work to block out noise.   If asking for a separate office is not feasible, you can try to work from home as much as possible to solve some of these issues.

5. ORGANIZATION, UNDERSTANDING INSTRUCTION

As mentioned before, some adults with AS find it hard to organize and understand information unless presented in a very logical and explicit way. Information and instructions have to be presented very clearly and often written down step by step. No assumptions can be made. An adult with AS will often be overwhelmed with an instruction to "get to work," look around them, see everyone working, and have no idea what they are supposed to be doing (and be too scared to ask), if information has not been presented clearly.

To deal with these organization challenges, someone with AS should start from the ground up and ensure that they understand what is expected of them. Many adults with AS get overwhelmed and are very reluctant to ask for specific direction. Asking a co-worker for specific advice may be easier than sitting down with your boss and may be the place to start.

Bring in a pad of paper and ask for specifics. Read back the instructions that you are given. Be very specific, which is relying on your strengths. After all, most AS adults are very good at focusing on a task at hand—as long as they know what that task is. Setting up a structured way of asking for direction can work. For each new assignment, set up a routine of asking what has to be done, what resources you are expected to use, when it is due and what the final deliverable should look like.

CAREERS THAT ARE BEST SUITED FOR ADULTS WITH ASPERGER'S

As mentioned before, adults with AS do have certain traits that lend themselves particularly well to certain fields.

Some of the things one should look for when looking for a job for someone with AS are the following:

- They are able to work as independently as possible (not a lot of team meetings or working with others)

- A career that requires attention to detail, patterns, or doing the same thing over and over (not right for all with AS , but fits many)

- Best jobs for people with AS: Computer programming, math, statistics, writing, languages, research, working in a library as a reference librarian, professor at a college, the arts if they are into this, engineering.

Worst jobs:

- Anything that requires constant interaction with people

- A job that requires things to be done under too much pressure

    o These could include having to work too fast or multi-task;
      especially a cashier, who has to interact with and perform a
      large number of things all at once while being friendly and
      communicating at the same time - speed, multi-tasking, and
      too much social interaction are *not* strengths of a person
      with AS.

PERSPECTIVE OF AN ADULT WITH ASPERGER'S

Some might wonder, what does it feel like to be an adult with Asperger's?
What does it feel like to be dependent on your parents for so much? How
do you feel about your future, your goals, your relationships with other
people?

Many studies, surveys and conversations have been conducted with adults
with AS on just these questions. Some of the most common responses that
emerged were the following. Adults with AS can often feel confused,
depressed and sometimes even hopeless about their increased dependency
on their parents even as they hit adult age. They feel like they should be
doing all the things their peers are doing, in the same way their peers are
doing them, and they don't understand why they can't, and why they seem
to fail so many times. Or, if they do understand, they just plain don't like it
and wish they could be more independent.

They may become angry, at their parents or at other people, for their lack
of abilities in this area. They may feel angry that society is constructed in
such a way that they can't seem to function fully and independently in it,
or depressed because they know they don't measure up to what society
expects of them.

Because Asperger's is an invisible illness, that is, not obvious from the
outside, many people with AS have experienced discrimination from
people who think they "should be able to do" a lot more than they are able
to do, which only feeds their feelings of inadequacy.

115

If the parents also do not understand why the child is having so many problems functioning in society, that can only compound the problem. Resentment can flourish on both sides, with the parents wanting the child to move out already and start supporting himself, the young adult wanting the same thing but not being able to do so, and having to deal with these feelings of failure.

The young adult wants to be independent, wants to prove to himself and others that he or she can be like everyone they see on TV, like their friends, in short, like a "typical 20 something year old," but because of the way their brain is wired, without a lot of support and creative thinking, it just doesn't work.

Support and education are the foundations for independence

With the appropriate supports and education about Asperger's, though, the child can often live independently and have a life of their own with only minimal support from their parents or other people who can help support them; however, until that time comes, or the appropriate supports can be secured, it can be a difficult time. The adult with AS wants to have a life of their own, stretch their wings, so to speak, but can't seem to succeed in any of the social arenas of life.

At the same time that they are struggling with having to be so dependent on their parents, they are often struggling with their social relationships as well. Quite often the adult with AS will come off as self-centered, insensitive, or just plain weird. It may look like the person with AS is not aware of how they come off, but they usually are; they just have no idea what to do about it. Or, as is usually the case, they are often not aware they have said or done the wrong thing until they get a bad reaction; then they realize that they goofed up, but they have no idea what to do about it, or how to repair the situation.

Adults with AS have a lot of anxiety about social situations for this reason; they are enormously frustrated that they cannot seem to connect socially, know they are doing something wrong, but don't know what. A good counselor may be able to gently help the adult figure out where they are going wrong and how to interact in a way that will be more likely to gain them the reactions and interactions that they desire.

One adult with AS put it like this while she mused over the question, "I try so hard to say and do the right things. Sometimes a conversation will start off right, and I can feel a connection with the other person, feel like I am doing it right.

They seem interested in what I am saying, and the conversation flows somewhat. Then all of a sudden I will say something, and the tone of the conversation shifts so abruptly, I can hear the disinterest and annoyance in the other person's voice. They stop sounding enthusiastic. They say they have to go. And I'm mentally kicking myself, having no idea what I just did wrong, wishing I could take back whatever it was and just start over, or at least know for next time so I can not do it and keep the conversation going for longer. Or, I think, was it my fault, and did the person really just have to go? Am I making too much of this? How do I know?" So, as you can see, even simple social interactions can be immensely confusing and frustrating for the adult with AS.

It is important for the adult with AS to focus as much as possible on their strengths, interests, and the things they CAN do to get them through this period of time until a more satisfactory way of life can be found; or, if this is the best they can do, to try to find some way to come to terms with and accept it as much as possible.

Again, some adults with AS are able to make the transition from high school and living with parents to college and the work world with relatively little difficulty and without needing a lot of additional support from their parents; it all depends on the individual person.

Different adults with AS have different goals. Some dream of college, getting married, getting a good job and settling down, just like everyone else. Some dream of a quiet room in a quiet house where they can, as one person put it, "be surrounded by nothing but textbooks and empty notebooks to write my ideas in all day."

Some have no idea what to think or dream about; they are either too focused on solving their present dilemmas or problems, or are just clueless about what they want, as are many people at this age.

Others dream of a day when they will have friends, be included in things, and not feel such an acute, painful sense of longing and loneliness; some just hope they will be able to find a job that allows them to be self-sufficient and take care of their daily living needs.

Some want to follow a dream, like to make art or move to England or do comedy shows. Some want to get married, some don't. Like everything else, the dreams and goals of a person with AS are different, but one thing is for sure: adults with Asperger's do have hopes and dreams for the future just like we do; they sometimes need to be modified a little, but they are hopes and dreams nonetheless.

Adults with Asperger's can contribute many positive things to our world. We need more people with this level of honesty and sincerity in the world. We need more people truly passionate about what they do, people who are able to truly enjoy and get excited over the small joys in life. We need people who can grasp, articulate, and solve serious problems, both of a technical issue and otherwise, without getting bogged down by small talk, petty arguments, or other social distractions.

In the population of our world, everyone has their own strengths and difficulties, and everyone is different and valuable in their own way. Adults with Asperger's are the same way; they have their challenges, yes, but they are definitely worth getting to know and having as friends and employees in the end.

An Asperger's Syndrome Guide

Bonus Report

Helping Your Aspergers Child Cope with the Holiday Season
By Craig Kendall

The sparkling lights of the Christmas tree. The smell of fresh baked gingerbread cookies coming out of the oven. Christmas carols on the radio, family you haven't seen in ages bustling in and out of the house. What could be better than the holiday season?

A whole lot, it turns out, for those with Asperger's Syndrome. While we may find many things to enjoy about holidays like Christmas, Hanukkah, Thanksgiving, and birthdays, someone with Asperger's Syndrome (AS) can get very frazzled by the disruption of their routine. Your child with AS may have many meltdowns and behavior problems during the holidays that are hard for you and others to understand. What can you do to help minimize these problems? In this guide, I will show you how to recognize the problem areas that come from kids with AS and the holidays, and many steps you can take to prevent and resolve them.

HOW A CHANGE IN ROUTINE CAN CAUSE HAVOC

First of all, you have to realize that kids with AS live on routine. Most of them want to get up at the same time, eat the same thing for breakfast every day, catch the school bus at the same time, watch the same TV programs, and so on. Their entire sense of safety and security comes from doing the same things every day. Now, when you have a holiday, everything is disrupted. There is no school, for one thing. People get up later. People don't do the same things they would do on a school or work day. While the change in schedule is refreshing for some, it can be miserable and scary to an AS child.

> **Their entire sense of safety and security comes from doing the same things every day.**

Secondly, you have to take into account the sensory issues that most children with Aspergers have. The Christmas lights on the tree will be too bright for them; the music will be too loud; the people will overwhelm them. Too many people moving about will be confusing and chaotic. They might not know what to say when relatives try to talk to them. They won't know when things start and when things end—in other words, they can't plan their day.

EXPECTATIONS OFTEN CAUSE CONFUSION

The expectations of the day may confuse them greatly. One thing that will set off a lot of kids with AS is opening presents. What is the appropriate way to react to a present someone has given you? When is it time to open them? When is it their turn? What if you don't like what you got? Some may even be bothered by the sound of the crinkling wrapping paper, and be overwhelmed by so many people surrounding them and expecting them to react.

If the family gathering, whether it be Christmas, Hanukkah, Thanksgiving, a birthday celebration or any similar get together, is taking place in someone else's house that is unfamiliar to the child, this might further cause anxiety, as the child is not used to the place.

Furthermore, for kids who have food allergies, there will be an abundance of food around that most likely they cannot eat. Either their intake of this food needs to be closely monitored, or special food tailored to the child's needs has to be prepared or taken with you.

So, as you can see, there are a wild variety of factors that can influence an Aspergers child's emotional state during a holiday gathering. This can result in emotional outbursts and unpleasant meltdowns just when you are trying to enjoy yourself most. Your child may throw a tantrum, refuse to participate, and embarrass you in front of company. This is not pleasant for either you or your child.

FORTUNATELY, THERE ARE WAYS TO AVOID THESE PROBLEMS.

The number one way to help your Aspergers child get through the holidays is to prepare him or her in every way possible for what is going to happen.

You need to tell him, "First, we're all going to get up around 8am, and then we're going to make eggs for breakfast. After we've had breakfast, we will gather around the tree for presents. You will open your presents first, one at a time. Then the other members of the family will open theirs. After this, we will...." And so and so forth, filling in the details for your individual family. Tell the child what the planned activities for the day will be, approximately how many people will be there, how loud it will be, and so on. Give him a sense of what to expect. Also, give him an escape route. "If it starts to get too loud for you and there are too many people, you can go in your room until you feel better."

Make sure you have reasonable expectations for your child. Do not expect him to be able to stay the whole time for a noisy celebration; let him take breaks in a quiet area. If you are visiting someone else's house, ask ahead of time if there is a quiet area your child can go to if he needs a break.

How detailed you need to be in these explanations depends on your child. Some will need more details than others and some will not need quite as much; you know your child best.

TRY USING A SOCIAL STORY

One useful way of accomplishing the above is the use of something called a social story. Simply put, you take a notebook, and on every page you write, in order, what is going to happen the next day.

Many people choose to illustrate these to give the child a visual image of what they will be doing. So, there might be a picture of the child getting out of bed, and the clock on the wall telling what time it is; and a picture of the child opening presents with the words, "I will be calm and wait my turn while I am opening presents. If I am upset by the noise, I can leave and go to my safe room." Again, preparation is key. The advantage to having it in book form is the child can look over it again and again and be reassured by knowing what is going to happen.

Tradition is very important to the Aspergers child. If you have always done something a certain way, it is best to continue doing it in that way in order to avoid problems that may arise for your child in breaking tradition.

SENSORY ASPECTS

Okay, so we've covered the importance of giving your child a sense of

> **If a meltdown does occur, take him aside and to a quiet area, and speak to him soothingly.**

what will happen during the day. Next, we will talk about the sensory aspects. It is important to try to keep the sensory aspects of the day as minimal as possible. In other words, if you have to play music, play something soft and soothing. Music can be very overwhelming to some people. Try not to invite too many people at once if you can help it. Reduce the visual clutter of the room the celebration will be occurring in, by storing the presents in one corner of the room or another room until it is time to open them. Be aware that the more sensory stimulation there is, the more overwhelmed your child is likely to get. If you see him looking a bit frazzled, perhaps you could pull him aside and ask if he wants to go to his safe (quiet) room.

Remember, if your child does have a meltdown, that it is not his fault. He is not trying to do it to make you mad. He is not trying to ruin your holiday. Getting angry at him will only make things worse.

If a meltdown does occur, take him aside and to a quiet area, and speak to him soothingly. If there are calming methods you have established that work to relax your child, use those. Empathize with his feelings of distress. "It sure was loud out there, huh? I bet that made you feel really overwhelmed!" or "It was hard to figure out what to say to Grandma and Auntie when they kept talking to you at the same time, huh?" Let your child stay in the room until he calms down, and then ask if he wants to rejoin the party.

A child might simply be distressed because something was done in the wrong order than they expected, and they don't know how to adjust themselves to deal with the disappointment of the new thing happening. In this case, it might help to point out the positives of the new situation, and tell them that what they expected is still basically happening, but with some modifications.

An example is a child who has been looking forward to cutting the first slice of birthday cake. Maybe they chose the cake specially and have been waiting all evening for it and to hear people's reactions to the cake they chose. But, for some reason, they miss the beginning of cake eating time, and burst into tears because they missed people's reactions to the cake they so painstakingly chose.

One thing that is important to consider is your own expectations of the holidays and your Aspergers child's participation in it.

They also did not get to cut it, and what's more, might be afraid everyone will eat it before they get a slice! Again, these things might not occur to you or me but definitely do to the Aspergers mind. In this case, you would make sure to praise their choice of the cake in front of them and tell them what a good job they did picking it, give them a slice, and focus their attention on how good the cake tastes, and not what they missed.

ASSESS YOUR EXPECTATIONS OF THE HOLIDAYS

One thing that is important to consider is your own expectations of the holidays and your Aspergers child's participation in it. You will get a lot more out of it if you keep your expectations at manageable levels. For instance, not expecting your child to be present the whole time, not expecting or pressuring him to enjoy it or say that he is enjoying it, and not making him talk to every guest that attends, are all things that will go a long way to improve the day.

Presents can be a challenge for all holidays. Often times the Aspergers kid does not know how to react to a present and might say something inappropriate, like expressing dislike for a gift, or saying that what they really wanted was some other model. They also may have trouble choosing what to open first, and just be overwhelmed by the general chaos of present opening.

One way to avoid this is to open presents ahead of time in private, so that way the child can take his time to look at the presents and react in whatever way he feels like it. Then thanks can be given to the gift givers at a later date.

You may want to warn other guests that your child may need to take a break from the festivities, may not feel like talking, or may have trouble with present opening time. This way, everyone can be prepared and no one will be surprised if slight social deviations occur.

THE KEY IS DOING A LITTLE PREPARATION

The idea is not to change everything about your celebration to such a degree that you or your guests do not enjoy yourselves. The idea is just to do a little preparation, so your Aspergers child can get just as much enjoyment out of your holiday party as you do (but in their own way). By following these tips, you will be well on your way to making the next holiday season one that you will truly remember!

An Asperger's Syndrome Guide

Bonus Report

The Aspergers Survey
of Parents and Professionals

Methodology and Conclusions

METHODOLOGY

- A survey of parents who had children diagnosed with Asperger's syndrome was begun in August 2008.
    - o Parents with children under the age of 21 qualified.
    - o Respondents were recruited from various internet discussion groups about Asperger's syndrome.
- Below are results from 106 respondents who completed the entire survey.

CONCLUSIONS

Diagnosis

- The results identify a major concern about the difficulty and length of time that it takes to diagnose Asperger's syndrome in children.
    - o While many children began showing symptoms by age 4, most were not diagnosed until years later (average age 11).
    - o Nearly half of the parents indicated that they had originally either been given an incorrect diagnosis or

that the diagnosis was clouded by multiple diagnoses or a diagnosis that was a long time in coming.

- o This shows the difficulty in getting your child correctly diagnosed and explains some of the reasons that it often takes many years before a correct diagnosis can be correctly made.

- o The most common person to make the final diagnosis was psychiatrist (35%) and pediatrician (30%).

  - ▪ Others mentioned included: neurologist, psychologist, councilor, family practice doctor, and child behavioral specialist

- o The most commonly mentioned early warning signs include social challenges (30%), focused on one subject / obsessions (30%), lack of eye contact (17%), sensitivity to noise/touch etc. (15%), and slow to begin talking (11%).

Causes of Aspergers

- The actual causes of Asperger's syndrome appear to be a mystery to many. Roughly half indicated "don't know/not sure" about two possible causes of Aspergers -- genetics and vaccines.

  - o Roughly one in three believes that Aspergers tends to run in families, while another third said that the cause of Aspergers may be vaccines.

  - o An issue making a correct diagnosis challenging is that many of those surveyed said their child had another diagnosis *in addition* to Aspergers.

  - o Most children received some type of vaccination prior to exhibiting signs of Aspergers.

    - ▪ While this, in and of itself, does not prove that vaccinations cause Aspergers, 1 in 4 parents believe that vaccinations are a cause (25%), and another 1 in 2 are not sure.

Medications

- Over half of the parents indicate that their children have been prescribed some type of medication for Aspergers.
    - Interestingly, no single medication predominates and a wide variety of medications have been prescribed.
    - Slightly more than half of the parents rate the medications that have been used to treat the symptoms of Aspergers as either "Very effective" or "somewhat effective."
    - However, 28% indicated that the medications were "not at all effective" and another 15% indicated that the medications "made symptoms worse." This points out how unique each case is.
    - Given the difficulty in arriving at a correct diagnosis for Aspergers along with the multiple diagnoses that Aspergers children often receive, parents should ensure that their physician has not arrived at a hasty diagnosis before allowing their child to take medications.
    - Many parents mentioned negative side effects of medications. Since no single medication was used by a large number of parents, we cannot draw conclusions about individual medications.
    - Overall, slightly less than half of the parents would recommend any medication. It is likely the parents who had some success with medications are the ones recommending medications to others.

Education

- Of the children in grades K-12, half were in a regular classroom.
    - Of the remainder, roughly a third are in a classroom for children with special needs, a third are home schooled while another third indicate some variant of these.

- 6 in 10 indicate that their child has an IEP (Individualized Education Program) at their school while another 1 in 10 indicates that one is currently being developed.
- In general, there is a high level of satisfaction with their child's school system.
  - 45 % indicate very satisfied while another 38% indicate somewhat satisfied with the school system.
  - Only 8% indicated very dissatisfied with the school.

Common Accommodations Made by Parents

- The most commonly mentioned changes to household routines to accommodate a child's needs are:
  - Sticking to strict schedules / routines
  - Maintaining structure
  - Counseling
  - Consistency with discipline
  - Dietary changes

Other Issues

- Roughly half of parents told their child that they had Aspergers between the ages of 5 and 10.

1. **Which of the following best describes your relationship with the child with Asperger's syndrome? Are you...**

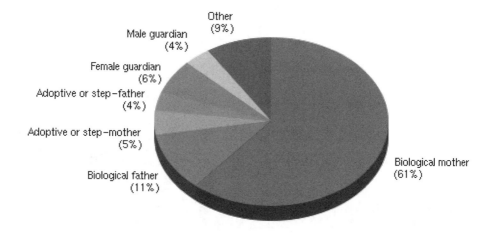

Other
(9%)

Male guardian
(4%)

Female guardian
(6%)

Adoptive or step-father
(4%)

Adoptive or step-mother
(5%)

Biological father
(11%)

Biological mother
(61%)

2. How old is the child with Asperger's syndrome? If you have more than one child with Asperger's syndrome, please answer these questions for the OLDEST child who is under the age of 21.

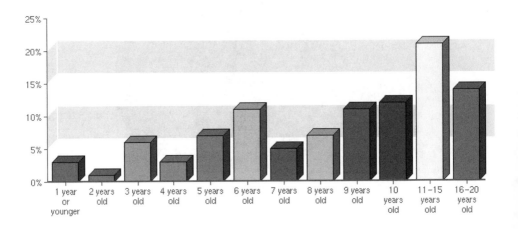

3. At what age did you first suspect that your child may have symptoms that concerned you?

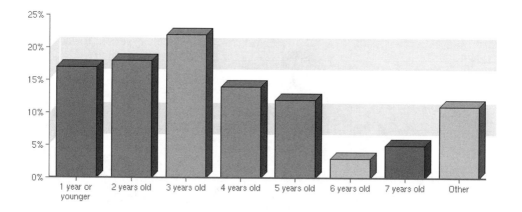

- **Average Age is 3.6 years**

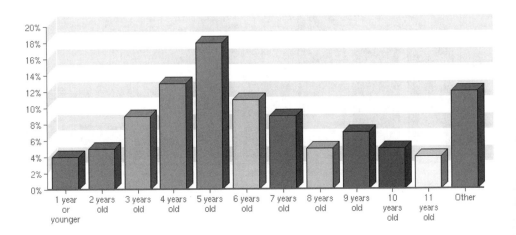

- **Average Age is 10.7 years**

- **While symptoms were first notices at an average age of 3.6 years, on average these children were not diagnosed with Aspergers until an average age of 10.7 years.**

- **It took nearly 7 years, on average, for a final diagnosis to be made from the time symptoms were first noticed.**

5. Does your child have Asperger's Syndrome in addition to another behavioral condition? If yes, what is the other condition?

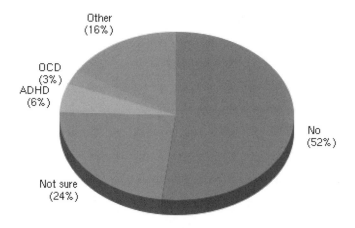

Other
(16%)

OCD
(3%)
ADHD
(6%)

No
(52%)

Not sure
(24%)

- One issue that may account for the length of time it takes to get a proper diagnosis is that children with Asperger's syndrome often exhibit symptoms of other conditions. Nearly half of the parents in the study either indicated that their child had another behavioral condition or they were not certain.

OTHER BEHAVIORAL SYMPTOMS MENTIONED	PERCENT %
Sensory Integration Dysfunction	2%
A.D.H.D	1%

ADD	1%
Adhd, OCD, ODD	1%
ADHD, OCD, PTSD	1%
AHDH	1%
Anxiety, panic disorder, Adhd	1%
mood disorder	1%
My Son also has ADHD	1%
Obsessive Compulsive disorder	1%
OCD, ODD, ADD, ADHD	1%
possibly ocd	1%
post traumatic stress disorder (anesthesia awareness)	1%
SI	1%
Tricholomania	1%

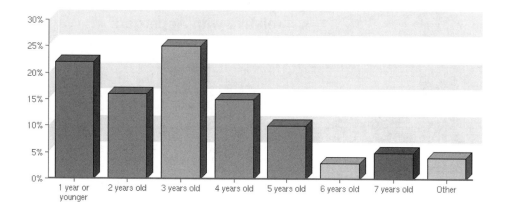

7. Are there any other blood relatives that also have Asperger's syndrome? (Select all that apply)

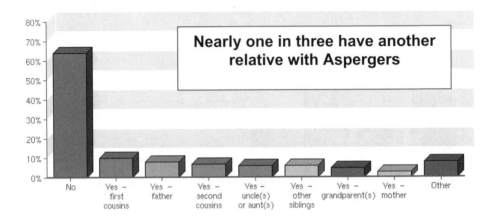

Nearly one in three have another relative with Aspergers

8. In your opinion, is Asperger's syndrome genetic? By this we mean does it tend to run in families?

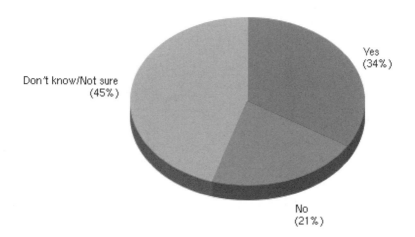

- **Roughly 1 in 3 believes that Asperger's syndrome's cause is genetic and another 45% are not sure.**

- **This is not surprising given that 1 in 3 families with an Aspergers child have another relative with Aspergers.**

9. Did your Aspergers child receive any vaccinations PRIOR to exhibiting signs of Asperger's syndrome?

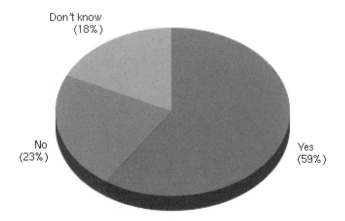

Don't know
(18%)

No
(23%)

Yes
(59%)

10. In your opinion, is there any causal relationship
    between vaccinations and the onset of Asperger's
    syndrome?

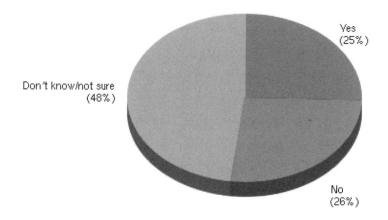

- **Most children received some type of vaccination prior to exhibiting signs of Aspergers.**

- **While this, in and of itself, does not prove that vaccinations cause Aspergers, 1 in 4 parents believe that vaccinations are a cause (25%), and another 1 in 2 are not sure.**

11. How old was your child when you told them that they had Asperger's syndrome?

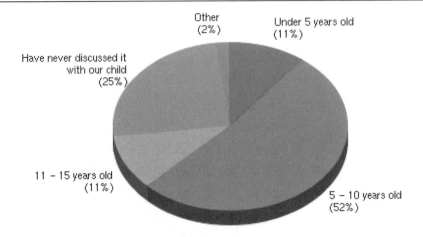

12. What medications, if any, have your doctors prescribed to treat Aspergers?

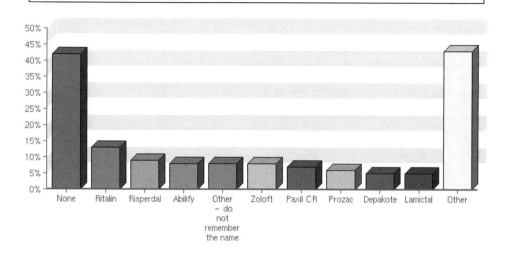

MEDICATIONS MENTIONED	PERCENT %
Ritalin	13%
Risperdal	9%
Abilify	8%
Zoloft	8%
Paxil CR	7%
Prozac	6%
Depakote	5%
Lamictal	5%

MEDICATIONS MENTIONED	PERCENT %
chlorpromazine	3%
Luvox	3%
Seroquel	3%
Topamax	3%
Zyprexa	3%
Anafranil	2%
fluphenazine	2%
haloperidol	2%
haloperidol (Haldol)	2%
Lexapro	2%
Geodon Oral	1%
risperidone and olanzapine	1%
Adderall	1%
ambien	1%
celexa	1%
Clonidinge	1%
for high anxiety but was only on 6mos	1%
lithium	1%

MEDICATIONS MENTIONED	PERCENT %
melatonin 2.5 mg nightly for sleeping	1%
Naltrexone	1%
right now we changed her diet and it seems to be very helpful	1%
STRATARRA	1%
Straterra, Vyvance	1%
strattera, but it was for ADHD	1%
Thorazine, Clonazapam, Celexa, Methylin, Naltrexone, Clonidine, Trazadone, Melatonin,	1%
Vyvance and its working beautifully	1%
We have tried a more natural approach with supplements and vitamins.	1%
Other – do not remember the name	8%

13. Please rate the effectiveness of each of the medications that you have used to treat the symptoms of Aspergers.

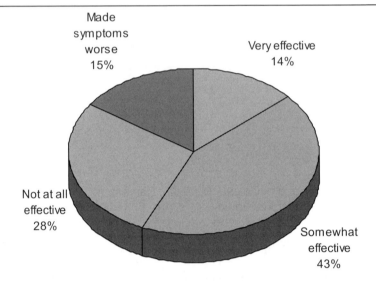

- Overall, slightly more than half of the parents felt that the medication their Aspergers child took was at least somewhat effective.

- However, only 14% felt that the medication was very effective while an equal percentage said that the medications made the symptoms worse (15%).

- Given the difficulty in arriving at a correct diagnosis for Aspergers along with the multiple diagnoses that Aspergers children often receive, parents should ensure that their physician has not arrived at a hasty diagnosis before allowing their child to take medications.

14. For each medication that you have used were there any negative side affects?

Below are listed medications for which parents mentioned negative side effects. Because no single medication was prescribed for many of the children, the results should be viewed as directional only. The side effects listed are just some of the possible challenges that these and other drugs may pose. Note: not all parents mentioned a side effect and some found these drugs very useful.

Abilify

- anger and aggression got worse
- Joint pain was complained of
- many

Depakote

- Rash, hyperactivity
- really sleepy when first started the meds

Geodon Oral

- weight issue

haloperidol (Haldol)

- affects appetite

Lamictal

- EYE EFFECT
- facial rash when combined with Depakote

Paxil CR

- it amplified her noise intolerance

Prozac

- 5mos after use-became dizzy and upset stomach
- made worse or same
- sleepiness

Risperdal

- he was very drowsy and dull but calm
- loss of appetite
- made more aggressive

Ritalin

- CRYING TICKS
- decrease in appetite
- Lack of response. Very tense.
- lost weight & sleep (adhd)
- Made him angry, jittery, and it changed his personality
- Made him irritable
- spaceyness
- wouldn't eat or sleep

Seroquel

- Extreme morning drowsiness/sedation
- weight gain

Zoloft

- gained weight
- stomach aches loose stool

Other

- adderal-loss of appetite, unable to sleep, twitches/tics
- adderal was horrible made him zombie-like and had no positives at all and he had no appetite

15. Which of the following prescription medications, if any, would you recommend for someone suffering with Asperger's syndrome?

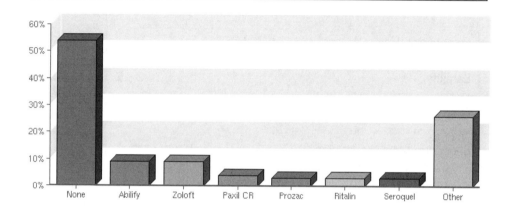

- Overall, slightly less than half of the parents would recommend any medication. It is likely the parents who had some success with medications are the ones recommending medications to others.

MEDICATION	COUNT	PERCENT %
None	50	54%
Abilify	8	9%
Zoloft	8	9%
Paxil CR	4	4%
Prozac	3	3%
Ritalin	3	3%

MEDICATION	COUNT	PERCENT %
Seroquel	3	3%
Depakote	2	2%
haloperidol (Haldol)	2	2%
Lamictal	2	2%
Luvox	2	2%
risperidone and olanzapine	1	1%
Anafranil	1	1%
antianxiety if it applies to them	1	1%
chlorpromazine	1	1%
clonidine to sleep	1	1%
diet change such as no caffeine more whole grains fruits, etc	1	1%
focalin or adderall (adhd)	1	1%
haloperidol	1	1%
I know other parents who have had success with Paxil and Zoloft.	1	1%
Risperdal	1	1%
Straterra	1	1%
Topamax	1	1%

MEDICATION	COUNT	PERCENT %
Vyvance	1	1%
Zyprexa	1	1%

16. How old was your child when you told them that they had Asperger's syndrome?

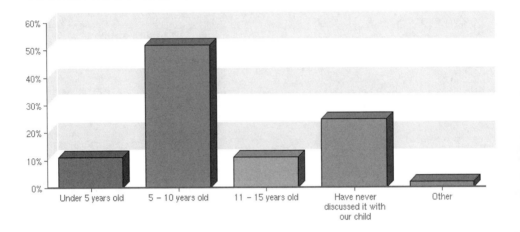

17. Is your Asperger's child currently in K-12 grade?

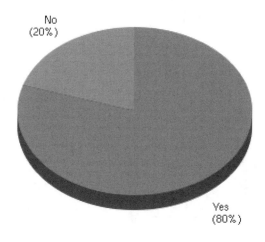

No
(20%)

Yes
(80%)

18. Which of the following best describes the type of classroom environment your child is in?

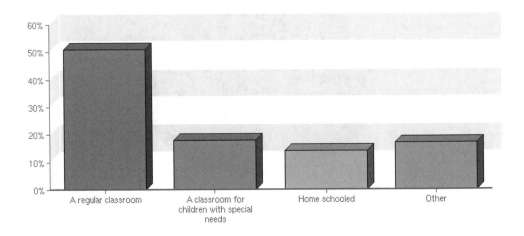

OTHER RESPONSES
1/3 regular, 2/3 special needs
3 hours a day in special education.
a classroom for ASD children with mainstream involvement as much as he can tolerate
A classroom for gifted & talented children
a multi aged class room with 1-3 grade (he is in 2nd) and its the perfect mix he gets along with the younger children and learns from the older ones its amazing, he does take all his tests with the special ed teacher
Autistic
both special and regular

He is in both special needs as well as normal classes
He is in resource for English, but AP and honors math and science
mixed preschool NT/spec needs
Public school with IEP and a school coach
regular & special with a 1 to 1
She was in special needs for part of the day, regular ed part of the day
small class of 10 students, 2 teachers
Special Ed with some standard classroom involvement
special needs class room with intermittent hospital homebound instruction
technical HS with "tracks" or "levels"

19. Does your child have an IEP (Individualized Education Program) at their school?

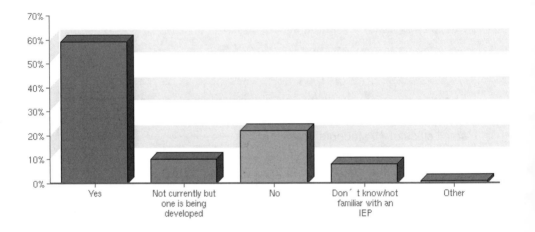

20. How satisfied are you with how well your child's school system has met his/her special needs? If not applicable (not in K-12 grade) leave blank.

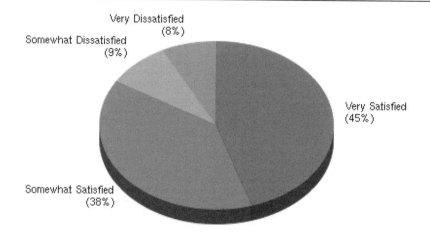

Very Dissatisfied
(8%)

Somewhat Dissatisfied
(9%)

Very Satisfied
(45%)

Somewhat Satisfied
(38%)

21. Did your child receive an incorrect diagnosis before finally being diagnosed with Asperger's syndrome? If yes, what was the earlier or incorrect diagnosis?

Yes, I originally received an incorrect diagnosis	25%
No	52%
Not sure	24%
	100%

- **Nearly half of the parents indicated that they had originally either been given an incorrect diagnosis or that the diagnosis was clouded by multiple diagnoses or a diagnosis that was a long time in coming.**

- **This shows the difficulty in getting your child correctly diagnosed and explains some of the reasons that it often takes many years before a correct diagnosis can be correctly made.**

LIST OF EARLIER INCORRECT DIAGNOSES LISTED BY PARENTS
ADD, bipolar disorder
ADD, Tourettes Syndrome, Bipolar-Mood Disorder-NOS, PSTD, LD, Autistic Tendencies
ADHD

LIST OF EARLIER INCORRECT DIAGNOSES LISTED BY PARENTS
ADHD
ADHD
ADHD
ADHD
ADHD
ADHD only.
ADHD, but overall our doctor was quick to realize that was *not* it.
ADHD, not sure at this time if he has it or not. Meds for ADHD do help, so he remains on meds for this.
At 2 1/2 my son was diagnosed with sensory issues and "something else".
At about 3 years old it was suggested that he had ADHD.
At first it was just ADHD with ocd -- then we saw another dr. that narrowed it from "autism" to Aspergers.
autism
autism
Autism and Developmental Delays
Can't say. Still trying to understand the complexity of the problem.
Disruptive Behavior Disorder - NOS
Earlier dx PDD-NOS and SI, not incorrect, just incomplete.

LIST OF EARLIER INCORRECT DIAGNOSES LISTED BY PARENTS

He was diagnosed with being mentally retarded.

He was diagnosed with many things from ear infections to adhd. I still go to doctors who say it's all in my head sometimes.

I suspected autism as her older brother has it, but never got her evaluated until after she graduated because the diagnosis would not have changed the outcome of her schooling plan. She was classified as "learning disabled," and had IEPs every year.

I was told there was nothing wrong with my child by our family doctor at that time.

mild autism

Most doctors said that Ryan had Autism

No diagnosis was attempted

No, but her kindergarten teacher didn't believe that there was anything wrong with her and dismissed my concerns. She described my child as extremely, extremely shy and either incapable of doing the academic work or simply refusing to do the work.

No, she was originally diagnosed with other things, but they also still remain on her list of diagnosis.

Obsessive Compulsive Disorder Oppositional Defiant Disorder

OCD, ODD, ADD, ADHD and inconsistent structure and discipline.

Original diagnosis was PPDNOS at just over 1 year old.

pdd nos which not necessarily incorrect just not specific enough

Reactive Attachment Disorder

She was first diagnosed as Selective Mutism disorder

LIST OF EARLIER INCORRECT DIAGNOSES LISTED BY PARENTS

She was thought to be mentally depressed

speech delayed autism pdd-nos

The doctor thought my child had hearing problems.

The earlier provisional diagnosis was PDD-NOS.

They always felt that he was somewhere on the spectrum, but did not want to label him unnecessarily. They also felt though it could be ADHD.

They said she was throwing temper tantrums and holding her breath.

Told he had quirky behaviors that he would outgrow.

We were originally told that his motor skill development troubles were simply due to his prematurity.

We were told he had learning disabilities at age three, and was given ot, and pt.

yes add and slight retardation

22. How was the initial diagnosis of Asperger's syndrome made?

INITIAL DIAGNOSIS

A neurologist made the initial diagnosis during an exam for CSE/Kindergarten.

A specialist for mental disorder diagnosed it after taking repeated psycho-analytical tests.

ADHD

ADOS

After 1 years worth of internet research on my part. I took my information to Dr. Appt. She referred us for testing.

after answering lots of questions by us the parents and the teachers at school

after being followed and examined by several experts

After discussing his behaviors and concerns with the pediatrician they mentioned that he had all of the markers for Asperger's.

after many appointments, had the school system helping quite a bit thanks to preschool

Akron Children's Hospital

at Emory Autism Center via my family doctor whose sister is autistic

At Hospital

Autism

INITIAL DIAGNOSIS

Behavior Diagnosis

By a child psychologist

By a psychiatrist

by a specialist

by DR

By elementary school Psychologist,& then a community Psychiatrist

By her pediatric psychiatrist on a routine visit.

By his school

By psychiatrist

By so-called evaluating my son when he first started school (kindergarten). I had never heard of it until they diagnosed him.

by testing behavior

Child Psychologists

Diagnosed by Aspergers Clinic, by watching him and questions.

Doctor

Doctor

Doctors ran series of test, months long after giving us the run around

Doctor sat us down and told us what she thought it might be and Saira (our daughter) went through a series of tests.

early intervention

INITIAL DIAGNOSIS

Erratic behavior

extensive evaluation by a child psychologist

Family Psychologist.

First a teacher suggested we get him retested.

Grandparents concern over behavior around other children.

He asked my son questions & watched him for a long time. the dr. had done extensive research on the subject

He hasn't been tested yet

his dad and uncle has it and he acted a lot like them

His doctor evaluated him, noticing very little eye contact, he also shows no empathy. He has a hard time socializes with other children.

His pediatrician took our concerns about his sensory issues and echolalia, suggested it might be Asperger's, and referred us to a specialist.

I am not completely sure. When I met his mother he already was diagnosis with it

I had to take my child to a special doctor out of town, since there are no specialists in my area.

I took him to his pediatrician because he seemed to dislike things he once loved. Didn't like going anywhere or trying new things.

inability to react

Interview

It became obvious by professionals

INITIAL DIAGNOSIS

It is very difficult to my son

My child was not making eye contact and he had no social skills when we put him in preschool

My husband and I searched the internet looking for what could all his symptoms add up to? when we stumbled on Asperger's it all fell into place and I talked to our doctor who after looking into it further, said it all made sense to him as well.

my mother noticed his behavior familiar

My son happened to be in a class where the teacher had a family member with Asperger's when he had a "meltdown". She suggested maybe having him tested.

My son was having a lot of trouble in school and we were tired of it being labeled ADHD, as the medications didn't work and actually seemed to worsen the problems.

myself, special educator

neurological and genetic assessment

neurological and genetic assessment as well as tests for cognition, psychomotor function, verbal and nonverbal strengths and weaknesses, style of learning, and skills for independent living

Neurological testing, hearing, vision, observing him in a school setting, observing him in social settings, complete physical (many), the ADIR, the ADOS, extensive psychological testing

Neuropsychology

Our child would get very upset at the slightest change in routine or his surroundings.

Pediatric Psychologist

INITIAL DIAGNOSIS

pediatrician

pediatrician

pediatrician

psychologist

question and answer

Ryan's psychiatrist and pediatrician performed some tests and came to the conclusion that he had Asperger's syndrome.

Sarah was acting out at school, and started skipping school all together.

School counselor recommendation for testing.

School psychiatrist

School Psychologist

School psychologist.

school testing

Series of interactions with psychologists

Still waiting on test results

team evaluation

Team of psychologists and psychiatrists

Testing at regular check-up

The first person to mention Asperger's to my husband and I was our son's developmental therapist.

INITIAL DIAGNOSIS

The initial (I call provisional diagnosis) was made by a clinical psychologist.

The school psychologist gave his teacher and I a questionnaire on AS to fill out and he scored off the charts. Then I took him to his pediatrician who gave us a referral to a psychologist.

There really wasn't an initial diagnosis (nobody wanted to make the diagnosis but I was referred to a developmental pediatrician).

They did a 4hour test at a CARE center.

This summer

Though a special place that does this sort of testing.

Through an extensive five-month long psych-ed assessment.

Through cognitive and physical exams.

through counseling and fast track at school

Through Early on Program

Through Pediatrician

through tests

Through the school

Thru Psychiatrist.

too painful

Took her to a psychologist, had an MMPI2 done, then took her to a special clinic dealing with memory and cognitive disorders.

took him to child psychiatrist

INITIAL DIAGNOSIS
VERY TOUGH IDENTIFY
we had a private psycho-educational assessment
We met with a doctor who did an IQ test and evaluated him for Asperger's.
With a pediatric doctor
working with a pediatric neurologist, school district and a CA regional district

23. Who made the final diagnosis (pediatrician, councilor, psychiatrist, etc.)?

PERSON MAKING FINAL ASPERGERS DIAGNOSIS	PERCENT
Psychiatrist	35%
Pediatrician	30%
Neurologist	9%
Psychologist	9%
Councilor	4%
Family practice doctor/physician	3%
Child behavioral specialist	2%
Pediatrician & psychiatrist	2%
Other	6%
Total	100%

24. What were the early warning signs that pointed to Asperger's syndrome in your child?

The following table summarizes the early warning signs that parents listed as pointing to Aspergers. Following this table are the actual responses typed in by the parents.

EARLY WARNING SIGNS THAT POINTED TO ASPERGER'S (SUMMARY OF RESPONSES)	PERCENT
Social challenges	30%
Focused on one subject / obsessions	18%
Lack of eye contact	17%
Sensitive to noise/touch etc.	15%
Slow to begin talking	11%
Extreme logic / spoke very proper / odd speech	9%
Bad behavior / aggressive / hit other children	9%
Needed routine	9%
Appeared lost / in own world	8%
Flapping hands	6%
Communication problems	5%

EARLY WARNING SIGNS THAT POINTED TO ASPERGER'S (SUMMARY OF RESPONSES)	PERCENT
Insomnia	4%
Stimming behavior	3%
Odd facial expressions	3%
Motor skill problems	3%
Could not sit still in school	2%
Sorting / separating items	2%
Other	19%

EARLY WARNING SIGNS THAT POINTED TO ASPERGER'S (VERBATIM COMMENTS)

Abnormal speech behavior.

Abnormalities like verbosity; abrupt transitions; literal interpretations and miscomprehension of nuance; unusually pedantic, formal or idiosyncratic speech

acted like she was in her own world, wouldn't look at others, didn't talk until later

antisocial

Antisocial behavior, rage, no participation, licks the TV, obsessive.

EARLY WARNING SIGNS THAT POINTED TO ASPERGER'S
(VERBATIM COMMENTS)

Anxiety and abnormal behavior.

At five years old went to relatives homes and wanted to see vacuum cleaner and explained all parts. Uncoordinated, weird body movements like tics and no eye contact, anti social.

At six months he would wake up and say good morning. Regardless of whether or not vaccinations play a role, after his MMR, he was a different person.

Autism is a complex brain disorder that affects many aspects of child development, including how a kid talks, plays, and interacts.

Avoiding eye contact Strange facial expressions Very delayed motor skills Was very over sensitive to loud noises

change of behavior

coughing

Could not follow or remember simple tasks, would not speak with anyone, could not concentrate.

Delay of developmental mile stones, stimming activities, fixation on one topic or item for hours, over sensitive to sensory stimulation.

Delayed motor development

EARLY WARNING SIGNS THAT POINTED TO ASPERGER'S
(VERBATIM COMMENTS)

Didn't really talk until age 3, Didn't like socializing with other children. Head banging when upset. Picky about what foods he would eat, sensitive to tags in clothing. Became a little professor about subjects that interested him, became computer literate at age 4 downloading files off the internet and putting them into his own files. Trouble with loud noises and light sensitivity. Does not like to be a large group of people this will cause a meltdown. Likes only non fiction. He feels fiction is not worth remembering he likes facts.

Difficulty making friends, difficulty with discipline, difficulty in the classroom, getting kicked out of three day care centers

Difficulty with social Interaction, obsession with things that were not normal for his age.

Dislike any changes in routines

Extreme Tantrums, Obsessive behaviors

Had speech, but echoliac. had hand flapping at an early age, perseverated severely, but then seemed to outgrow a lot of it

Halted social development.

Hand and arm flapping, ritualistic type behavior, limited interests, social awkwardness, lack of empathy at times, trouble sleeping, sensory issues.

Hand flapping, tantrums, no affection, no eye contact, didn't play with toys, spun around in circles a lot.

Hated changes in daily routine, not very socially interactive.

EARLY WARNING SIGNS THAT POINTED TO ASPERGER'S
(VERBATIM COMMENTS)

He couldn't get along with anyone. Including his mother or myself. And once his mother moved she was sure that something was wrong.

He has obsessive interests (Thomas and Friends is EVERYTHING.) He is VERY regimented in his routines down to which sock goes on first, can't stand dirty hands, etc. He gets over stimulated VERY easily and has frequent melt downs in high sensory situations. He "talks to himself a lot" and attaches to objects such as taking a movie case with him everywhere. He also speaks in a peculiar manner for his age.

He used to get unnaturally upset if there was any kind of change in his surroundings.

He was a low birth weight baby despite being full term. He had a birth defect which was found after birth and required surgery. He was given many meds. in the nicu. because of this I watched my son very closely, and after about his 9th month and several ear infections, he started to not keep up with what i expected him to be doing for a child his age. Did not wave, clap, point, did not respond well to his name. etc

He would often avoid eye contact even when you are speaking directly in front of him. He often would have these odd facial expressions that just did not seem typical.

His lack of speaking things he should at his age. he also flapped his hand a lot. He just didn't respond like we felt he should to things.

Hyperlexia lack of "play" language very formalized routines and speech - scripted speech.

I always thought she lacked social common sense and was socially withdrawn.

EARLY WARNING SIGNS THAT POINTED TO ASPERGER'S

(VERBATIM COMMENTS)

I didn't know anything about Asperger's before the diagnosis. However, the symptoms that concerned me were his inability to work independently at school, his poor handwriting, and the fact that he has always just seemed uncomfortable in his skin, so to speak.

I honestly didn't have a clue, I was new to it. I thought the way he acted was from the ADHD. After speaking with his psychiatrist and his evaluation, he told me about the disorder and to research it. I then realized after reading about the disorder, that yes my son does have it.

If I had known- He didn't sleep (really) for the first 2 years of his life. He always seemed out of sorts. He was so smart he was doing high school math in 1st grade.

Impaired language development, stereotypical behavior, etc

In Pre-k her teacher constantly wrote notes home saying she seemed 'sad' and she rarely interacted with the other children and her use of words was different than the other kids.

Inability to communicate with people effectively

insomnia

Lack of eye contact, fussy, unable to focus, couldn't walk until 2.5 yrs of age.

lack of eye contact, seems to be in his own world, uses extreme logic, sensitive to noise and touch......

Lack of eye contact, unresponsive to name, single-minded focus on certain objects (construction vehicles, Thomas the Tank Engine, cars)

EARLY WARNING SIGNS THAT POINTED TO ASPERGER'S
(VERBATIM COMMENTS)

Lack of focus. Isolation.

lack of speech

Largely, it was that he only repeated things that were said in the script from his favorite computer game.

Loner type behavior, loud noises making him irritable, sorting and separating toys food etc. strange behaviors in general. Friends/ family comments.

Low activity, odd behaviorisms

Meltdowns in public situations, hypotonia, oral aversions, tactile defensiveness, lack of eye contact.

Mostly communication problems. Not able to have a back and forth type of conversation. Also, the earlier testing showed that his processing speed was above normal.

Motor skill/dexterity problems, clumsiness, hand flapping when he got upset, inability/unwillingness to interact socially

My child acted differently than other children and he did not seem to be developing normally.

My son was not hitting the usual baby milestones. He stopped developing physically at the age of 6 months.

Needed constant motion while awake, being in a baby swing, thought he had a hearing problem, he was way behind by age 2, early intervention people came 3 times a week.

no eye contact

no eye contact, melt downs, black/white thinking

EARLY WARNING SIGNS THAT POINTED TO ASPERGER'S
(VERBATIM COMMENTS)

NO one listens to me all noises, people, clothes texture problem and more bothered our child.

Not being able to express love, very aggressive, does not pay attention

not liking certain clothing, bad behavior, not caring about discipline, getting on one subject and never getting off

obsession, routine, good with math

Odd behaviors, antisocial, developmental delays in some areas but very good at reading and obsessed with crop circles.

Off in her own little world. EXTREMELY sensitive to stimulation, especially with noise.

Our child avoided eye contact, had very strange facial expressions, needed to have a very stable routine in which he became very upset when it was changed, was very un-empathetic, had many one-sided conversations as he began to talk/advanced his speech which is not at all how myself or his father speak.

Poor attention span in school and lack of desire to socialize with other children

Repetitive and intense abnormal behaviors

Repetitive stacking/playing and attention deficit

rigidity, bizarre behaviors (flapping, etc.), unusual and consuming interest in specific things, lack of interest in peers, low eye contact, poor communication skills,

EARLY WARNING SIGNS THAT POINTED TO ASPERGER'S
(VERBATIM COMMENTS)

Ryan was very clumsy, he was never able to make friends with other children, he'll walk up to strangers and start conversations, a lot of times he'll pick something out about a person like that they like Obama, and he'll go up to them and just be negative about Obama and promote McCain even though he knows it's going to hurt their feelings. He was overly violent which was weird because we never promoted that in the household.

Seizures

Sensory issues showed themselves as early as 24 hours old, though we weren't thinking Asperger's at the time; we were told he would be an 'intense child'.

She didn't begin talking to age 4.

She exhibited odd behavior at a very young age. When she was approximately one year old, she would become hysterical if we did not take the same route to and from her daycare. She would become so hysterical that she was able to force her way out of the straps of the car seat and wedge herself above the backseat by the back window, screaming "Wrong way! Wrong way!" She didn't like to be hugged. Sounds, smells and textures would cause her to become very upset and sometimes to throw up. She wanted to be friends with other children, but when unknown children would approach her, she would stare straight ahead and pretend she couldn't see or hear them. She didn't know the names of the other children in her kindergarten class until 8 months into the school year. These are just a few of the things we noticed.

She was very slow in her activities, and was not able to make friends in play school.

Similar to hyperactivity at early ages. Once beginning school we learned that noises bothered him. He would sit and cry, put his hands over ears and rock himself.

EARLY WARNING SIGNS THAT POINTED TO ASPERGER'S
(VERBATIM COMMENTS)

sleep issues, sensory issues, OCD type behaviors, fixations, perseverations, anxiety,

social & emotional challenges, exaggerated emotions, stims, (twitches or tics) did not know how to play with peers(parallel play) appeared "lost" a lot

Social situations. Meltdowns!

social skills

Social Skills, strange obsessions.

Socializing with others, constant movement, sensitive to smells.

speech delay behavior eye contact lacking apraxia

Speech delays and social delays.

Spoke very proper, didn't look in your eyes

staring blankly while unable to communicate

stimming behaviors, difficulty in social settings

Temper, speech, not doing well with others

The assessment commenced due to what appeared to be dysgraphia.

They (the school) said because he wouldn't sit still, didn't follow directions and hit other kids when he wanted something from them but he couldn't express himself.

EARLY WARNING SIGNS THAT POINTED TO ASPERGER'S
(VERBATIM COMMENTS)

tip toes, Thomas the Train (excessive); lines things up, didn't talk till he was 3, pointed and grunted at things.

too much pain

Unable to participate in any group activities, unable to carry on a conversation outside of his interests.

UNNECESSARY TALKING

Unusual language usage and patterns, not socializing in what I considered to be a normal way, very odd mannerisms, would get overly upset if his routine was at all altered

Very black and white, advanced vocabulary, could build well with instructions - put together toys, Transformers, Legos, etc. , very little eye contact, in his own world often, ...

We noticed our child was not making any friends. He was too shy. He would have almost obsessive patterns to how he would do things. They had to be done that way or he would not be able to function.

withdrawn behavior

Would not look me in the eyes ever.

25. What specific Asperger's symptoms does your child exhibit?

ASPERGERS SYMPTOMS CURRENTLY EXHIBITED

when diagnosed(at 7 yrs old)... exaggerated emotions, immaturity, unable to make & keep friends (did not know how to make friends), socially uncomfortable, preferred to be around immediate family & adults, or very young children. Did not know how to socialize around peers. My child is 16 now & most of the symptoms appear to have slowly resolved themselves

poor social skills, stimming, poor fine and gross motor skills

tips toes walking even at 14, Thomas the train (love of); blow outs, excessively immature for his age -- fascination with clocks/time

He started reading at very early age. hyperlexic. He sometimes talks obsessively about topics of interest. Very poor social skills, seems very anxious sometimes.

Not sitting still.

lack of sleep

Hard to make friends, overly obsesses over odd topics or objects.

Difficulty with social Interaction, obsession with things that were not normal for his age. Obsessive compulsive, strange quirks

He sometimes talks much of the time, and it's often about the same subject over and over. And he lots of times speaks whatever thoughts come to him. He does not censor himself.

Talking about one subject a lot, abnormal behavior in social situations, avoiding eye contact

ASPERGERS SYMPTOMS CURRENTLY EXHIBITED

Upper body rigidity, minimally reciprocal social interactions, restricted areas of interest, executive function impairments, exceptional intelligence

Bothered by sounds. He does not understand correct things to say at the times. He is kind of obsessive compulsive about things. He is a loner, has an odd gait when he is running and he is extremely smart.

routines, perseverations, anxiety, fixations, socially inappropriate

Mainly his expressions and reactions to others in his speech.

He flaps his hands a lot, and makes a sound while doing so. He doesn't do things (typical) he should for his age. He has to ask to do almost everything. Social grouping is not typical. He seems to be in his own world.

social skills, nervous tics

social skills language delay behavioral lag ocd

Behavior and context of situations.

Lying, routine, obsession with horses and other animals, likes food to stay the same.

Intense preoccupation with a narrow subject, one-sided verbosity, restricted prosody and intonation, and motor clumsiness

Impaired language development, stereotypical behavior, etc

Social, sensory (hearing & touch), speech, and strong interest and skills in math and music

hands over ears, not looking at people and not social

ASPERGERS SYMPTOMS CURRENTLY EXHIBITED

Loud noise reactions, needs food separated on his plate so it doesn't touch. Fascination with things that turn into obsession, stays in his room to play alone for endless amounts of time. Does play with friends but only video games, unable to ride a bike or show interest in it. Has taken a coin jar and made a beautiful design out of it on my carpet. Runs out in front of cars at age 10, must be held on to in parking lots. Unable to let him walk around in a store, if he feels separated from me or other adult panics. Needle stick are a source of horrible panic attacks, he turns purple and thinks he will die from a blood draw.

Cannot tolerate certain noises, has meltdowns with stress, cannot stay focused on tasks, and yet can get "stuck" on other tasks. Needs encouragement to move from one task to another.

Mild social problems now. Different way of looking at things. strong desire to be "normal"

speech, anger.

aggressive, not showing love, inattention

Touch ADHD, OCD, PHOBIA, learning disabilities.

Seizures

poor motor skills, still can't run right and he is 10. he has no social skills, he get over stimulated easy. he can't cope with stress of any kind good or bad it's all the same to him. He is so smart, at things like math, but the concept of thinking for him self needed in English is just too much for him. He can't write an original sentence to save his life. I'm sure there are more but right now that is the best I can do.

Tantrums, odd compulsive behaviors

Isolation. Narrow range of focus. Affected speech.

black/white thinking, occasional melt downs

very shy, doesn't like sudden routine changes

ASPERGERS SYMPTOMS CURRENTLY EXHIBITED

hates any change

Little eye contact, basically ADD, black and white concepts, difficulty writing and putting thoughts on paper, lack of imagination, excels on his interests - math, reading. Attracts younger friends. Not interested in sports. Competitive with mind games, puzzles, math, etc. Not social unless he's showing off his Transformers collection. Will not start a conversation. We have to ask 50 questions to find out what he did in a given day at school. Hygiene could be better - doesn't wash or rinse hair well - needs reminders. Picky eater. Won't ask questions if he needs help.

coughing

with 7+ years of weekly pt, ot, speech, vision therapy, and craniosacral therapy, my guy is doing fantastic, though by 'normal' standards, he's still not social, and not adjusting well to the new school year.

social withdrawal, flapping, OCD

awkward social skills, difficulty making friends or knowing how to act in a given social situation, obsession with video games and video game characters, and inappropriate voice inflection.

Sensory issues inability to read social cues very high intelligence needs reliable routine language delay.

unusual facial expressions

Obsessive behaviors, Tantrums, Anxiety, Social

anti social behavior, rage, no participation, lick the TV, obsessive

She continues to play with the same toy all the time. She cannot write neatly how much ever she tries.

o c d anti social

ASPERGERS SYMPTOMS CURRENTLY EXHIBITED

Insensitive to hot and cold, gets them confused. Must have routine, no routine, severe behavior, tantrums. Will not look at you when he is talking to you or when you speak to him, yet he is very bright.

Little eye contact. No empathy trouble socializing totally fixated on one thing and doesn't care if no one else likes it. His verbally skills are good although he takes things in the literal sense.

She gets frustrated with people and wont talk to people she considers beneath her. She has difficulty understanding other peoples emotions, and reasons behind their actions. She also cannot see there are consequences to her actions unless she does it.

avoids eye contact, talks about one of his favorite objects

abnormal psychological behavior

laughs too loudly and too long very outgoing, less aware of how welcome he is hard to get along with same-age peers, does great with adults and little kids

abnormal speech

Most particularly, she will not speak with anyone she is not 100% comfortable with, so she will not connect with teachers. She is not able to stay on task but has a very high IQ

He's an exceptionally talented musician, he's also quite clumsy and he has been obsessed with cars since he was very young. He can name every make and model for any car that exists. He is a very bright boy.

Most prevalent is the social ineptitude

ASPERGERS SYMPTOMS CURRENTLY EXHIBITED

Social anxiety and lack of social skills. She wants to have a friend but doesn't know how to make a friend. Hyper sensitivity to sound and smell. She doesn't like to be touched. Seems to be advanced academically for her age, but her social skills fall behind. She has severe problems with making transitions. She becomes frustrated and then hysterical quite easily over seemingly inane things such as the toothpaste is crooked on her toothbrush or there is too much or too little water in the glass. She assumes there is only one correct answer to any question, so if someone answers "good" instead of "fine" - she will become very agitated because "that's not the right way."

He has had extensive therapy since we have known about this for a while and he is fifteen. He actually attends a regular high school, has friends, and is quite normal.

He did not make eye contact and could not hold a two sided conversation. He is very smart and likes to tell you about things he knows, but cannot handle being interrupted. He also has a tendency to hold his hands in awkward positions when it is inappropriate

Social irregularities, too touchy feely with his peers, is book smart but not street smart, advanced way of speaking, doesn't use contractions when he speaks, has meltdowns, clumsy, overly sensitive, can't read the body language and cues from others, didn't have any friends until this past year.

Poor socialization skills

rigidity, difficulty with social interaction, abnormal interest in very specific things

Aversion to touch, occasional echolalia, sensory issues when it comes to clothing.

fixation still an issue as well as sensory issues

Socialization problems, advanced speech patterns, easily over stimulated by environmental factors.

Repetitive and intense abnormal behaviors

ASPERGERS SYMPTOMS CURRENTLY EXHIBITED

See above. He now also obsesses on subjects such as Pokemon, planes and WWII and will talk about them even if you are not listening.

Does not socialize well with other children. Has trouble with loud noises and can not stand when more than one person is talking because he can not understand what the people are saying, trouble writing, depression, does not like to be around large groups of people. Feels the weight of the world is on his shoulders and he wants to make it better but does not know how.

Autism symptom exhibit causing delays in many basic areas of development such as learning to talk and interact with others.

Social Problems. Changes is daily routine

Communication problems, speech impediment, over focusing on certain topics.

Lack of eye contact. Disconnect with peers. (Now verbal) Odd speech- not appropriate at times.

no eye contact, arranges colors

He has obsessive interests (Thomas and Friends is EVERYTHING.) He is VERY regimented in his routines down to which sock goes on first, can't stand dirty hands, etc. He gets over stimulated VERY easily and has frequent melt downs in high sensory situations. He "talks to himself a lot" and attaches to objects such as taking a movie case with him everywhere. He also speaks in a peculiar manner for his age. He has even adopted the British slang from Thomas and Friends.

odd behaviors, mechanical like movements,

See above.

Social, social and social (lack of skills). Depression.

echolalia, rapid hand movement, mood changes, ignores the world outside of his realm

ASPERGERS SYMPTOMS CURRENTLY EXHIBITED

He's very clumsy, very awkward in social situations, and violent.

echolalia, trichtotillomania, sensory integration problems

antisocial

She mostly lacks empathy and social skills

same as normal

He is awkward in almost any social situation, usually functioning on the edge of any group, he will talk endlessly about videogames, he likes to twirl small straight objects near his eyes, he is kind of awkward physically.

very literal, clumsy, routine, smell and sound sensitivity

Communication issues, Speech Delay, Behavioral problems

Anti social, no eye contact, emotionally and developmentally slow.

Poor communication and repetitive behavior

zoning out, random outbursts

Motor skill/dexterity problems, inability/unwillingness to interact socially, obsession with planes, hand flapping, very fast talking

My child seems to be in his own world sometimes. He has problems dealing with people and has a strange way of communicating.

Trouble interacting with other children, dislikes changes of schedule, unusual facial expressions, talks a lot, and delayed motor development.

26. What changes have you made to your household routine to accommodate your child's needs, if any?

CHANGES MADE TO HOUSEHOLD ROUTINE TO ACCOMMODATE CHILD'S NEEDS

a morning schedule more structure I've become more aware of what his triggers are

A special teacher to manage and control her behavior has been appointed and she is specially trained to adapt to everyday life.

Additional counseling to understand certain behaviors.

Always encouraging play dates. give alternative behaviors to stimming

Begin getting ready for things earlier and spend more time discussing events with him

breakfast; lunch & dinner (are timed); med taking is exact; med's in containers so he remembers to take them.

dairy free, give warning of all changes

Diet, routines. Some visual aids.

disclosure of diagnosis

Easier walking access

Food separation, assignment of dining room chairs, strict meds schedule, harder to find babysitters that can deal with behaviors, harder to find playmates, difficulty with teacher accepting diagnosis, much much difficulty with 3 other siblings, more supervision than should be necessary for his age needed, dealing with angry outbursts. I could go on and on.

CHANGES MADE TO HOUSEHOLD ROUTINE TO ACCOMMODATE CHILD'S NEEDS

haven't quite figured that out

He has his own bathroom, computer so he can take his time doing whatever he needs to do. He is beginning foreign languages at school so I bought him several beginning language music CDs that have all the basics in songs.

He needs to have everything in order; every thing has its own place. We have to keep the house picked up.

healthy atmosphere and friendly environment

home schooling

Homework- setting a timer helps and we still sit down with him to do his homework. We do have a well organized and very routine life which seems to help him.

Honestly, not many. She is a picky eater so we try to meet those needs and we try not to change certain things, like never re-arranging her room furniture.

I guess routine is the key word. We just keep to it. Everything else is normal.

I had to accept a job at home to accommodate his care. Everything is done to make sure not to upset our household routine at all.

I have to rearrange things in a different way to suit my child and keep him calm and happy. My child follows a different diet than other family members.

I home school her, I talk to her and we do a lot of things together

I tried to help my sister adjust to having a job, and I tried to teacher her to drive, but she was unable to learn. She came to my house with a drug and alcohol addiction. I managed to get her to stop taking drugs, but she still drinks. She says it makes her feel normal.

CHANGES MADE TO HOUSEHOLD ROUTINE TO ACCOMMODATE CHILD'S NEEDS

I try to keep some kind of structure. Any change in his routine, will result in a meltdown. from his morning routine all the way to his bedtime.

just have given moral support and provided independent living conditions

Just having him calm down when he feels frustrated. Tried the Brushing Technique.

Just really stay with routine, etc.

just slowed down on how the house is run, take more time and not rushing

just try to keep things even keel for him.

keeping him in separate room when lots of people in house

Keeping on a strict schedule and explaining if something will be different, aside from the normal routine.

Largely creating a routine, *period*.

less spontaneity

maintain structure, work on social skills, and had him in a program through Hope Haven.

maintaining a consistent, planned schedule is helpful, being organized

Making changes would be the wrong thing to do in Saira's case. We have had the same routine since she was 2 and any change would pretty much destroy her perfect world. I recently gave birth to a baby boy (Nikolas) who is 4 months old now and that has been a huge change for her.

Mother's career goals and schedule, put off moving to a new home, changed schools, changed diet to non GMO, organic, changed to all natural non chemical household cleaners and products.

CHANGES MADE TO HOUSEHOLD ROUTINE TO ACCOMMODATE CHILD'S NEEDS

No change in routine because he doe not like change

Not many, as I still have so much to learn about Asperger's. I think the only real change I've made is that I'm much more patient while helping him with his homework. I know realize why it takes him so long to do it.

Our household revolves around Adam's schedule, needs, tolerances and abilities. His brother is his best supporter, and understands him and his needs better than most parents. Hard to say what we've done to accommodate him, pretty much everything. We consider him before we do anything, from practicing drums, to turning on the TV.

Our routine revolves around our child to alleviate any anxiety he may have.

Pic. charts, cut things out of diet

preventing him from seeing things that irritate him

Routine charts, advance discussion of routine and/or changes,

Routine, Routine, Routine,

run a schedule with everything we do

Schedule is more rigid, that is what he likes.

schedules

Schedules, repeating what "the rule" is, a lot, for many years until it finally sunk in. A lot of repeating things to my child until things sunk in

Special ed at school.

Started scheduling everything. Discipline methods changed. We used to not follow through on a lot of "if you don't quit I will do...." We learned that he needs to have that.

CHANGES MADE TO HOUSEHOLD ROUTINE TO ACCOMMODATE CHILD'S NEEDS

Strict medicine time and bedtime, basic schedule of when we eat, go for a walk.

Strict Routines

The way I discipline him. They don't understand punishment after the fact you have to get to them before they do something wrong. I try and make sure I have friends with younger children he can play with so he feels like he has friends (he gets along with younger kids a lot better) I try and stick to a regimented schedule so he has no surprises

Very few actually. He is doing very well in fairly "normal' conditions...

visual schedules, deep pressure input, head set for noise issues, pre prompting for changes

we are more consistant with discipline

We give him a wide berth so to avoid getting him angry. He for the most part eats what he wants because he won't eat everything, but what I give him is healthy. I am divorced from his mother and she feeds him and all the other kids junk food mostly. I'm still trying to get custody.

We had child that crashed and burned couldn't leave the home, was bullied at school. There is no burping in our home because in school everyone did it. No short sleeve shirts, Anyone that looks or reacts in certain way they cant come into our home.

We have a pretty structured daily schedule.

We have added visual cues where possible we try not to stray fro routine, even when something exciting is happening we created 'retreats' where our son can go to calm down.

We have been to a few different counseling sessions and have him medicated for ADHD which has seemed to help. We also have created coping mechanisms to help him with everyday tasks.

CHANGES MADE TO HOUSEHOLD ROUTINE TO ACCOMMODATE CHILD'S NEEDS

We have not made that many. We keep to schedule for meals, and bedtime, try not to over stimulate because melt downs still occur, but not as frequent. We have another son neurotypical, and we just do everything as a family.

We have tried to "slow down" and work around his temperament. We no longer "rush" to do things and try to allow plenty of time because we found that by telling him we were "running late" it only caused him to get more upset. We have tried to cut down/eliminate those items that we know send him on "sensory overload." We have altered his diet and we are still working at how to lessen/shorten the melt downs as well as what other things trigger them.

We help her with studying and do things.

We pretty much need to keep things calm around here. I tried babysitting my niece and nephew, ages 10 and 13, but my daughter got so agitated I just couldn't do it anymore. I work from home so that I can take her to appointments. She gets over stimulated easily, so keeping the group to a minimum helps. She likes to eat the same foods. Drives me nuts.

We provide warnings (30 minute, 10 minute, 5, etc.) when we know a transition is approaching. We have "do overs" as an opportunity to "go back in time" and make things the way she likes them. We don't raise our voice with her because that causes her to become highly agitated. Instead, we try to be silly and cajole her into calming down. We have her put a bit of salt on her tongue to keep from gagging and vomiting while she brushes her teeth.

we spend more time with him which my child need

we tend to follow the same routine, or sequence of activities, we have to be careful about transitions, make sure that preferred foods are available, he needs very close following to see that homework and other non preferred activities are completed well so use picture schedules at times

We try not to change any thing around him. I try to be with him as much as possible.

We try to keep the routine the same as much as possible.

CHANGES MADE TO HOUSEHOLD ROUTINE TO ACCOMMODATE CHILD'S NEEDS

we try to keep things the same, don't move furniture or anything he is used to

Well his mother moved not to long ago, but since I have met his mother we have not changed anything.

We're becoming more structured, to deal with her higher need for structure and routine.

We've found that structure is very important and spending a lot of one on one time.

We've taken away any movies, video games, or toys that promote violence. We try to speak softly. We have someone come to the house three times a week to help Ryan work on his social skills.

27. What changes or accommodations have you made that have helped the most?

CHANGES / ACCOMMODATIONS THAT HAVE HELPED THE MOST

Advanced warning.

all of the above....but still working on it everyday.

All. Diet, routines, visual aids

at one point I home schooled for 2 years. after a very difficult kindergarten year, my son made no progress, and seemed very immature as compared to his peers, so I home schooled for 1st and 2nd. and put him back in school for 3rd gr. it was still hard but is getting a little better. school still remains a big issue because of social etc.

Avoiding red food dye, due to symptoms of extreme behavior. Strict medication schedule, use of Zoloft at night, routine adherence, family cooperation and acceptance.

Being understanding and keeping calm

Calming him down when he got frustrated.

Counseling

Cutting down on TV and computer time, and spending lots of time, hugging and loving him.

dairy free, give warning of all changes

Definitely being organized and routine has helped him the most.

dietary and household chemical changes, giving up all pharmaceuticals, doing all natural biomedical/homeopathic treatment

CHANGES / ACCOMMODATIONS THAT HAVE HELPED THE MOST

Discussing issues and how to work around them

discussions and explanations help him

Easier walking access

friendly atmosphere

Gave him the master bedroom. Gives him room for all his stuff but gives him a safe place to get away from everyone.

Giving warnings - lots of preparation for even the slightest bit of change. Giving chance for a "do over" - seems to calm her down. Remaining calm ourselves even in the face of what seems to be the most absurd and frustrating situation. Not showing our frustration and anger.

has a dog companion trained for autistic children

He has a private tutor which gives him one-on-one time and this has helped him. Sometimes it can be overwhelming if he is around too many people at once.

head set is wonderful, looks unusual but is great for cutting out noise and getting the behavior response

hilly area

home schooling

home schooling him

household modifications

I am very strict, but very consistent and have a very specific routine.

I took a class on how not to yell at your kids when they stress you out and that has helped, and I also had to come to the fact that I am not going to be able to make him be able to do things.

CHANGES / ACCOMMODATIONS THAT HAVE HELPED THE MOST

If Sarah stays on a schedule and does the same thing everyday she is fine, but she can't handle changes.

including him in everything I can

independent living conditions

Just keeping a regular schedule for the whole family makes everything run smoother.

Keeping a controlled, calm environment has helped. The stability is key around here, and that is by her knowing someone trustworthy is there for her. Any stress we as parents are experiencing needs to be filtered because it affects her negatively. She gets really emotional, so we have to monitor what we say about what, where and when. Redirecting her into an activity that she enjoys calms her when she is upset. She has a snake, and that is key for her, too. Something about the movement of the snake around her hands calms her.

Keeping her routine the same is the biggest thing that helps her. We also got school involved in letting her know about fire drills, when the schedule was going to change, and they allowed her to leave each class early so that she would not be in the halls during passing period. She went to a very large high school and the halls were loud and very crowded. The school involvement helped tremendously.

Keeping routines as constant as possible

kept a schedule of things, try to interact with others

Learning what triggered his meltdowns and slowing life down. Trying to be more patient with him.

Minimization of upsets in routine, increased structure, increased social situations

more discipline

CHANGES / ACCOMMODATIONS THAT HAVE HELPED THE MOST

Mother ensures that he is active in sports and has made the sacrifice to place him in a very structured private school and he loves it!!!!

My staying beside him keeps him calm. And the thing that we have tried and it works to some extent is explaining to him about the possible change before hand

None really, we treat him as we would any of our other children.

none we are all treated the same in our home we don't want him to rely on pity to get through life we will be dead some day and he will have to take care of himself

Not going to large crowds, helping her develop friendship with a friend of mines daughter, they write and send packages to each other to another part of our state.

not straying from routine, even when exciting things are happening (i.e.: last minute party invite, staying up late for movie)

One change was to have a dog which helped our child a lot.

organization and structure

Our living room has been turned into a therapy room, with crash pits, swings, bouncy balls, bosu balls, etc.. We warn him before we make any unusual movements or noise (example: I'd never run the sweeper or blow dryer without warning him first) we have custom ringers on the phone that don't startle him, and got rid of the doorbell.

pick your battles more routine more advance planning for errands or other changes of routine

planning and scheduling things in advance so there are no surprises for him

play dates

Practicing social skills.

CHANGES / ACCOMMODATIONS THAT HAVE HELPED THE MOST

preventing him from watching certain TV shows

Probably just the help that we get from others; support is key.

Probably talking in a soft voice as my child does not like loud noises and is easily upset. Also changing my child's diet and eating more natural foods and less junk foods.

Putting him in charge of his own things.

Routines - knowing what is coming and making what is expected an automatic part of the day.

schedule / routine

Schedule adherence and listening to him.

schedules

Setting firm, non-subjective boundaries.

She has special facilities to create interests that benefit her overall social development, friends come home everyday to help her overcome her shyness.

She likes to be included with helping Nikolas such as making a bottle or simply washing his face off. But when these things happen they have to occur at the same time everyday or she simply seems not to care. It breaks my heart a lot of the time because I feel like somewhere beneath all of the stony features is another little girl I get to have seldom glimpses of.

sleeping environment

staying calm myself

staying to an exact time frame helps.. keeping the clocks exact also.. he has a fascinations with time

CHANGES / ACCOMMODATIONS THAT HAVE HELPED THE MOST

Sticking to routines

stopped going to work to spend more time with him

Study help

The most important change has been scheduling. My son seems to have better days when he has total structure and scheduling.

The schedule helps tremendously, If he gets off his routine it really makes for a bad day, and if he is surprised with anything(doctors visit, or apt) He gets very upset

therapy

Understanding his reactions more and watching his clumsiness. Trying to make the home safer for him.

Visual aids to help with appropriate social behavior.

We just work very hard with him, to improve on his skills etc. We give him lots of love and he responds well to that.

We no longer try to force her to speak with other adults or children. This has eliminated a lot of her anxiety issues as well.

We put him in a school that offers a low ratio classroom setting so that he gets more individual attention to help him succeed.

We try to keep everything simple. And not to seclude him in any way at all

We went and saw an alternative doctor that did an all natural heavy metal detox. We had results within days.

We've tried to consciously cut down on background noise.

What has helped him most that I have done is to listen to him more and to sit and talk to him more about things on an equal level.

***

The information presented in this book is educational and should not be construed as offering diagnostic, treatment or legal advice or consultation. If professional assistance in any of these areas is needed, the services of a competent autism professional should be sought.